AVID

READER

PRESS

Enough

Your Health, Your Weight,
and What It's Like to Be Free

ANIA M. JASTREBOFF, MD, PhD
OPRAH WINFREY

Avid Reader Press

New York   Amsterdam/Antwerp   London
Toronto   Sydney/Melbourne   New Delhi

AVID READER PRESS
An Imprint of Simon & Schuster, LLC
1230 Avenue of the Americas
New York, NY 10020

This publication contains the opinions and ideas of its coauthors. It is intended to provide helpful and informative material on the subjects addressed in the publication. Coauthor Dr. Ania Jastreboff, a medical doctor, provides content in this publication for general informational and educational purposes only, and it is not a substitute for professional medical advice, diagnosis, or treatment. This publication is sold with the understanding that the coauthors and publisher are not engaged in rendering medical, health, or any other kind of personal professional services in the book. The reader should seek the advice of his or her physician or other qualified health care provider with any questions about a medical condition or potential treatment and should consult with such a qualified provider before drawing inferences from any content in this book.

The coauthors and publisher specifically disclaim all responsibility for any liability, loss, or risk, personal or otherwise, which may be incurred as a consequence, directly or indirectly, of the use and application of any of the contents of this book.

Some patient names have been changed. Some patients represent composites of several patients.

Let's stay in touch! Scan here to get book recommendations, exclusive offers, and more delivered to your inbox.

ANIA M. JASTREBOFF, MD, PhD

For you.

If you live with obesity and have carried silent pain.

*May you find freedom through knowing that
obesity is a disease, not a choice.*

May you find hope, compassion, and healing.

We hear you.

OPRAH WINFREY

*To Julius G., Nicholas M., Derrick R., and all those who
struggle and have blamed themselves. May you find peace
with the knowledge that obesity is not your fault. No
amount of willpower can change your brain or biology.*

Contents

Enough

Preface

I have never felt better, stronger, or more fit. Even when I turned forty, and ran my first and only marathon, I didn't feel as alive and open to new exploration or as vibrant as I do now.

I hike. I bike. I take long walks. I do resistance weight training, even deadlifting, at least three times a week. I have parties for one where I dance and play on the lawn with my dogs. I now plan vacations based not only on the best food but on the best hikes. I go nowhere there isn't plenty of access to exercise. I hardly recognize the woman I've become.

It's taken me more than half a lifetime to get to this point of freedom from worry, blame, and shame for a body that persisted in holding on to more pounds than I felt comfortable bearing. I now understand why. The cause was biology! My trying to fight being overweight all these years was as futile as my trying to fight being five feet, six inches tall.

Only in 2023 did I learn that obesity isn't what I thought it was. It's not a size. It's not a number. It's not even a condition caused by overeating. It's a disease, one the American Medical Association recognized in 2013.

Somehow, I missed that memo and continued blaming myself for every pound lost and consistently regained. All these years I thought I could do it myself. And as the Lord and all his disciples know, I've tried and failed, tried and failed, tried and failed. In front of all of you, who have borne witness to it. The failure has felt doubly shameful because I have access to so much: chefs and trainers and the healthiest of foods.

Why couldn't I lose the weight and keep it off? Because no amount of success, money, fame, or intelligence is a match for biology. I had a disease and blamed myself for not being able to cure it. As one doctor I interviewed put it, "It's like holding your breath underwater and trying not to rise."

I did this for most of my adult life.

I remember back in 1985, I was thirty-one years old and invited to my first appearance on *The Tonight Show*. I was there to talk about my little talk show in Chicago that was beating the legendary Phil Donahue.

I had never been more excited or felt more accomplished. I splurged an entire week's salary on Stuart Weitzman rhinestone shoes. And I had a blue suede dress handmade by a local designer. It was a proud moment. My first time receiving national recognition for my little local show. Before we went live, Johnny Carson's producers had gone over all the topics we would discuss. They either didn't know or forgot to mention that the guest host, Joan Rivers, would create one of the most humiliating moments of my life.

I'll never forget the moment she looked at me and said, "How'd you gain the weight?"

I nervously laughed. "I ate a lot."

"No, no, no," said Joan. "You're a pretty girl and you're single. You must lose the weight!"

Joan went on and on, insisting I drop fifteen pounds immediately—sooner if possible, ideally right there onstage, wearing my specially made blue suede dress. I was, of course, surprised and flustered. I tried to explain that I was trying to lose the weight and that I would lose the weight. We ended the conversation shaking hands, agreeing that I could come back on the show if I lost fifteen pounds.

For years, until recently reviewing the clip on YouTube, I'd thought she'd actually said, "Shame on you!" Because that was all that was echoing in my mind, sitting there in my rhinestone pumps. She hadn't! I had made up those words for her. And worse, I *accepted* that I should be shamed. I thought, "She's right . . . How dare I be sitting up here on *The Tonight Show* at this size?" I left embarrassed, humiliated, but surprisingly, not angry. Because I agreed with Joan! She was right, in my mind. I didn't deserve to come back until I was thin.

Soon, it became public sport to humiliate me. I was literally a running joke. David Letterman made fun of me for an entire year. It wasn't just late-night comedians who wanted an easy joke at my expense; the tabloids tracked my ups and downs better than any Fitbit. Every week they made money off shaming me with headlines like "Oprah Fatter Than Ever," "Oprah Hits 246 Pounds: Final Showdown with Stedman Sends Her into Feeding Frenzy," and "Oprah Warned: 'Diet or Die.'"

I blamed myself. I tried every weight-loss trick in the book. I was always on a diet, off a diet, on a diet: the cabbage diet, the watermelon diet, the fruit fast, where you just do nothing but a different fruit every day, the Atkins diet. I remember one where you were supposed to eat only green things, no white things.

For decades, the shame of not being able to manage my weight took up so much space in my brain. I tried everything and yet nothing worked. I was convinced that I just needed more willpower.

Because it hadn't always been like this. Growing up with my grandmother, we had a little farm in the back of her property down in Kosciusko, Mississippi. We raised our own chickens, grew our own vegetables. The meals were simple and delicious. Back then food meant you were prosperous enough to have it. But years later, when I moved to Baltimore, I had to eat alone in my kitchen. For company, I would walk over to the mall and "shop" for dinner at the food court. First I'd visit the baked-potato bar with all the fixin's. Then the salad bar, with more fixin's, heavy on the bacon bits. Then the chocolate chip cookie stand.

From the outside, I'd made it—I was one of the city's youngest local news anchors. But on set, my cohost, Jerry Turner, was not happy to have me there. This middle-aged, white-haired anchorman was used to doing the show by himself and didn't want a twenty-two-year-old taking up his airtime. He made that *very* clear. I remember him asking me, "What school did you go to? Is that accredited?" Another time he said, "You're from Mississippi? Can you name all the tributaries of the Mississippi River?" I looked at him, feeling inadequate. Unbelievably, I thought, "I've got to go right home and memorize all the tributaries of the Mississippi River."

At home, after long days of this kind of belittlement, food became my solace, my comfort, my reward. I didn't realize I was using food to avoid conflict or sadness. I went to see my first doctor about my size in 1977.

From then on—for more than five decades—much of my life would be dedicated to fighting my weight. I had the success and the acclaim, but I still would gain . . . and lose . . . and repeat the cycle over and over again.

Years later I remember going with Stedman to a World Heavyweight Championship and the announcer saying Mike Tyson's weight—218 pounds. I was also 218. In that moment, I felt sorry for Stedman. Here's this beautiful, handsome guy, and he's with someone who weighs as much as the heavyweight champion of the world.

I was determined to do something about it—and I did. You may have seen the clip of me in 1988, pulling a red wagon with sixty-seven pounds of fat, to show how much weight I'd lost after four months of a meal-replacement diet. During those months, I'd canceled any events that had to do with food, including my first trip to Venice. Who can go to Italy and not eat? All to prove I could get back into a pair of size 10 Calvin Klein jeans.

Even though all the naysayers said, "You'll put the weight back on," I thought my four months of discipline would prove them wrong.

Within two weeks of stopping the diet, I'd gained back eight pounds. The star of *Miami Vice*, Don Johnson, invited me to his holiday party that year, but I stayed home, because I thought, "I'm too fat to go to his party." I was so disappointed in myself for gaining weight back. For letting it happen again.

Had I learned my lesson ten years later? No, I had not. When Anna Wintour suggested I lose twenty pounds before appearing on the cover of *Vogue*, I worked my behind off, literally. I did everything I could to get in shape, and it paid off. I was transformed into their October cover girl.

But then the weight came back.

I spent years like this, yo-yoing, trying and failing. "Why can't I just conquer this thing?" I said to myself over and over. "Why can't I solve this problem?" In 2009, I even appeared on the cover of *O, The Oprah Magazine*, standing next to my thinner self from 2005, under the headline "How Did I Let This Happen Again?" I thought, "Oh, if I say it myself, then other people can't say it." All I did was give everybody else the right to continue to judge.

I swallowed my shame. I accepted that I'd brought this on myself. The cycle continued.

In 2018, a friend mentioned they were taking a drug meant for people with diabetes that helped them control their weight. They said they could help me get on it—a shot to the belly. I said no. Number one, it's for people with diabetes, and I did not have diabetes. Number two, if I went on it, everybody would say I took the easy way out. I still thought my weight was my fault—and if it was my fault, I believed it was my responsibility to fix.

In 2021, I got my new knees. Grateful to be walking without pain, I started hiking religiously. I was up to five or six miles a day and eating one small meal at 4 p.m. I lost some weight. People started to comment. And I thought, "Maybe that's the answer—one meal a day and putting in the miles." Then the holidays came, and I still gained eight pounds. I cannot tell you how demoralizing that was. Here I was exerting all this energy, the mental load, the cognitive load of fighting the wish to eat. The battle was constant.

In 2023, I hosted a panel conversation with weight-loss experts and clinicians, called *The State of Weight*, as part of *Oprah Daily*'s "Life You Want" digital series. I had the biggest aha along with many people in that audience when one of the doctors said that in 2013 the American Medical Association had recognized obesity as a disease.

I realized I'd been blaming myself—and my lack of willpower—for years. It's not about willpower—it's about the brain!

Immediately after that conversation, I called my doctor and said, "You mean it's *not* my fault? I have something that causes this to happen within my body? Are you kidding me? Get me on the meds *today*!"

Within days, I noticed a change. We have the best English muffins in the world in our house. They're from this little place, the Model

Bakery, in Napa Valley. Before the medication, I could eat two of those English muffins without thinking—one with jam and then another with honey. Now I couldn't finish a whole one. I was satisfied with half. I'd had enough.

Something happens in your brain on the medication. You eat only when you're hungry, and you stop when you're full. I couldn't believe it.

This is what it's like to be free from the constant pull of food, I realized. Free from the constant chatter in your head about what to eat, how much to eat, how much you just ate, how many calories it cost you, and what it's going to take to burn off those calories.

An aperture had opened in my mind—I saw new possibilities. And I see them now every day. I say yes to life.

I no longer turn down invitations to parties or trips to Venice. I look back and understand why I made those decisions then—I felt ashamed of not being able to manage my weight. Even when I was first offered to take the shot, I was still feeling embarrassed I couldn't do it myself. But hear me when I say that life with these medications has ended the struggle with my weight. I use them as a tool to enhance all aspects of my health. Having the food noise go silent created a space for so much more. I now look forward to exercising without feeling like it's punishment. I move because it's easier for me and makes me feel so much better—not just physically but emotionally, mentally, even spiritually. I feel connected to myself. I feel whole. Doing a panel discussion on weight in 2024, I met Dr. Ania Jastreboff, an endocrinologist and professor at the Yale School of Medicine. She has been studying obesity for nearly twenty years and researching the GLP-1-based medications for a decade and a half. In this book, she answers the questions so many have regarding these medications. Dr. Ania shares story after story about the people with obesity who found these medications to be life-changing. She breaks down the science, the treatments, and, yes, the biology. Most important, she explains that the goal in treating obesity is not just weight reduction. It's about improving and optimizing your overall health. I can say amen to that.

—OPRAH WINFREY

My "why" in life is helping people with obesity. So when Oprah raised the idea of writing a book about obesity, the answer was clear. Together we wanted to share a truth. And that truth is that obesity is a disease. It's not a choice. It's not about willpower. It's a disease. For Oprah, as for many of my patients, this truth was a lightbulb moment. And embracing this realization changes the entire conversation around weight and health.

If you have obesity—the disease—it means that your body wants to store more energy, even if it already has enough to live, move, and exist. You don't just experience obesity in your body. You may experience it in your conscious and subconscious mind. It emerges as food noise, that relentless voice in your head urging, no, demanding that you eat another cookie or chip even after you've finished the whole bag. You may be constantly distracted by trying not to eat. That takes a lot of effort, focus, and energy. You may have tried diet after diet, trying to fight your own biology. All these behaviors are not you. They are symptoms of a disease.

So, part of my "why" is helping my patients understand that their weight and having obesity is not about fault or failure. And that's why Oprah and I wrote this book. To tell the truth about the disease of obesity. To describe the new treatment options. To set your mind and body free from fault or self-blame and, if you so choose, to lay open potential new paths for improving health.

I'm often asked where my "why" came from and how I came to do what I do. Let's start at the beginning. Unbeknownst to me at the time, I started on this path at a very young age. In the early 1980s, my parents came from Warsaw to the United States to further their research in molecular cancer biology and systems neuroscience, which they had started at the Polish Academy of Sciences.

With them they brought their two young children (me being one of them), a couple of suitcases, and not much else. As PhD scientists working at Yale, they did have one thing: their education. I grew up in a household where one of the first purchases they chose to make—even though finances were so tight that sometimes my parents borrowed money to buy food—was a set of encyclopedias for my brother and me.

Along with learning, food and tradition was a comfort, a central part of our lives through celebrations and holidays—pierogi, schnitzel, borscht, and bigos (hunter's stew). Our everyday meals were more simple—veg, starch, protein—as my parents couldn't afford more at the time, but we were never left wanting. Eating at restaurants was not a consideration. Even so, food meant love, and that was how our mother showed her affection for us. As my brother would say, "Forty thousand calories of love" at every holiday and all the days in between.

At ages six and eight, new to America, my brother and I attended public school although we didn't yet speak English. We grew up close, the constant in each other's lives, in the face of so much change. And that's why I will never forget how my older brother, whom I adored and looked up to, was teased as a child.

In middle school, we moved from a small city to a charming New England town populated by many generations of Italian and Irish immigrants. We were not from Italy or Ireland and, lacking money, often wore secondhand clothes and the same clothes multiple days in a row. We were relentlessly teased for being smart, for wearing clothes that were not cool, and, my brother, for his weight. His nickname became "Spanky" (from *The Little Rascals*). An introvert by nature, and highly intelligent, he taught himself how to read books every morning while walking to the bus stop (miraculously without tripping), instead of chatting with other kids.

One day he walked into a classroom and sat in a combo chair desk, and the chair broke. It was an old, rickety piece of furniture, and likely a coincidence, but that became a very embarrassing memory and moment for him because the other kids blamed it on his weight.

My brother joined the swim team in the seventh grade, and the weight began to come off. It wasn't until later in high school that he grew tall and transformed. But to this day, I think that in his mind, he still exists as Spanky. Seeing my beloved brother bullied about his weight never left me. His experience sparked my desire to help people with obesity.

My father is the next and main reason why I work in the field of obesity. Eventually my parents were able to afford more, and food became more diverse and abundant. Nothing was wasted, and anything extra was stored. The running joke was that there was enough food in our basement to feed us for several years if there was an apocalypse (so we playfully referred to it as "the nuclear bomb shelter"). As teens, when my brother and I had friends over, you never knew when my mother would "just" whip up a scrumptious oven-roasted turkey in the middle of the night, just in case we were hungry. She loved to cook and always made our favorite foods.

Over the years, my father slowly began to gain weight. Food had been scarce in his postwar upbringing, and he was taught to finish everything on his plate. Now in an environment of abundance and in the rewarding but fast-paced and stressful life of academic scientists, my parents traveled the world, and slept little, writing research grant proposals at all hours of the night. There was no bedtime; they worked until the work was done. Somewhere along the way my father developed obesity, and while I was in college he was diagnosed with type 2 diabetes. It was very hard for him to accept this diagnosis. He tried medications and diets. He felt guilty eating, knowing his blood sugars would rise. My mother, too, gained weight over the years, developing knee pain and high blood pressure. They both tried every diet under the sun—the cabbage soup diet, the DASH diet, the Mediterranean diet—and they'd lose weight, but then they would inevitably gain it back. My father's story had a powerful foundational influence on me, as obesity had significantly impacted his health and well-being. My entire family knew what types of food and how much we should eat, but all the education and new resources resulted in little when it came to weight.

I realized then, seeing my highly intelligent father's struggles, that a person could know what they *should* eat and yet be compelled by biology to do something else. At that time I did not yet understand that biology was driving his behavior, but I did know that carrying extra weight, storing extra fat, was not about choice. My father did not choose to have obesity. My mother did not choose to gain weight. My brother and I did not choose to have a genetic predisposition to weight gain, obesity, or diabetes. None of us chose to live in an environment that promotes unhealthy weight gain.

By coincidence, I loved running. In high school I began long-distance running, joining the cross-country team. The crunchy fall leaves under my feet, cool air blowing on my face, ponytail swinging—there was something so freeing about it. I quickly developed from the worst runner to one of the best. Then in my twenties and thirties I ran 10Ks and half-marathons, and in my thirties and forties, triathlons. Every year, weekends (and training schedules) would be structured around my favorite races—the Army Ten-Miler, the Cherry Blossom Ten Mile Run, the Rock 'n' Roll Virginia Beach Half Marathon, and the Iron Girl Columbia Triathlon. As a high school athlete I had become interested in the relationship between food and our bodies, and over time I grew more curious about food nutrition and its relationship to health, weight, and physical activity.

In medical school, among the hundreds of hours of lectures, we did not have even one presentation about obesity. It was the late 1990s and for the most part obesity was not yet understood to be a disease. Leptin, the first identified fat-secreted hormone essential for body-weight regulation, had just been discovered in 1994.

After many sleep-deprived nights, I earned my MD. My medical residency was also a blur, as we worked more than eighty hours most weeks. Nevertheless, I became fascinated by the countless endocrine feedback loops and how hormones, as key messengers in those loops, impact so many different bodily functions. Little did I know then that there were soon-to-be-discovered hormone loops and pathways between the body and the brain that would be key to understanding and treating obesity.

During this time I began to wonder why some people could eat whatever they wanted and never gain weight, whereas others seemingly ate very little, yet weren't able to lose any weight whatsoever. I went into my postdoctoral fellowship at Yale wanting to take care of people with obesity and hoping to better understand the biology underlying this disease.

My fellowship was in both adult and pediatric endocrinology.

I had an extraordinary mentor throughout my early years as a physician-scientist: Dr. Robert (Bob) Sherwin was a giant in the field of diabetes and endocrinology. Compassionate, intelligent, and incredibly generous with his time, he encouraged me to pursue a PhD in the neurobiology of obesity. During my PhD, he paired me with an extremely innovative neurobiologist and psychologist, Dr. Rajita Sinha. Among many other things, she had developed a way to better understand how people's brains responded to stress, and then adapted this to look at how people responded to food cues using a brain-imaging method called functional MRI. Together with several other investigators, we looked at brain responses to thoughts of food, pictures of food, and drinking sugar. My mentors, Drs. Sinha and Sherwin, left the door open for me to study obesity and understand how biology impacts behavior. Dr. Sinha also enabled me to start seeing patients with obesity clinically, when no obesity clinic existed at Yale and no one was focusing on obesity treatment and care.

I began avidly reading about obesity as well as attending lectures and conferences, finding steadfast support and guidance through senior faculty who were experts in obesity treatment at Harvard, Cornell, and other institutions. In those early days there were only a couple FDA-approved medications for the treatment of obesity (orlistat and phentermine); bariatric surgery was a treatment for those with more severe obesity, while lifestyle interventions were the predominant mainstay for most. It was during that time that I began seeing patients with obesity. I began listening to my patients and learning from their struggles, their successes, and their stories. They all worked incredibly hard. They were motivated and committed. They had grit. With few exceptions, they always gained back the weight, the weight that they dutifully lost time and time again. Over the years my research moved from brain-imaging studies to clinical trials with new medications. Eventually, with the support of our forward-thinking and intentional medical school leader, Dean Nancy Brown, the Yale Obesity Research Center—called Y-Weight—was created. As founding director, I lead landmark trials investigating new obesity medications and conduct research studies to better understand the biology of obesity. I share this knowledge with the general public as well as clinicians around the world through lectures and speaking engagements (and sometimes podcasts and panels with Oprah). I am incredibly grateful to find deep meaning and purpose in the work I do: caring for people with obesity, studying new treatments that have the potential to become approved medications, and then seeing how these new medicines help people worldwide.

So that in a nutshell has been my medical career path as a physician-scientist. But when people ask me why I do what I do—it's for the love of my family: my brother, my mother, my father. This is why I find so much meaning in taking care of people who struggle with their weight, who have obesity—why I feel joy when I help them understand the biology of obesity, when I help them find the treatment that's right for them, help them turn hope into reality, and begin to feel free from the relentless pull to store more energy. I never thought that having obesity was my father's fault, so why would I think it was any of my patients' faults? The answer was in our biology, all along.

The truth is, our bodies are brilliant! Millions of years ago, our bodies figured out that in order to survive, we needed to store fuel or energy, and that the most efficient way to do this was to store energy as fat. Fat is a good thing: It allows us to survive and thrive. We have this beautiful and essential biology whereby hormones communicate with our brains about energy needs and stores in our bodies. Our brains regulate these energy stores, making sure we always have . . . *enough.*

But for some of us, it's *never* enough.

No matter how much you eat, you're never full; you're always left wanting. In the back of your mind, there's always the thought of . . . the mint chip ice cream in the freezer, the rich and velvety fresh spring mangoes, or the crispy fries and perfect melty cheeseburger that's just an Uber Eats order away. Maybe you're not even conscious of this, but your mind is never clear. You're cozy at home watching Netflix, and somehow you find yourself wandering into the kitchen, opening the pantry without really knowing what you're looking for.

You may ask, if we have such vitally important biology, then why do so many people have obesity? Why does my neighbor have obesity? Why does my daughter have this disease? Why do I have it? Nearly half of Americans have obesity; two-thirds are overweight or have obesity. Certainly, hundreds of millions of Americans did not wake up one morning and choose to have a disease. Obesity is not a choice; it's confused biology. So what happened? Why do so many of us store extra energy, extra fat?

It turns out that our environment changed much more quickly than our biology evolved. The environment we live in is filled with ultra-processed food, lack of sleep, lack of physical activity, and a lot of stress. This environment promotes the storage of extra energy, and we respond by doing just that—storing extra energy, extra fuel. Our bodies are simply making sure that we have *enough.*

The patients that I see in clinic and study participants I see at Y-Weight are relieved to hear that having obesity is not a choice: It's not their fault; it's their biology at work.

I do not have obesity, so what I know, I have learned from listening to my patients and my trial participants: hearing their struggles, their successes, their voices. By sharing their stories, my patients have taught me so much. What it feels like to try and try and try to lose the weight, then lose it, and have it come right back on. What it feels like to never be satisfied, never be sated. What it feels like to never not be hungry—the minute you finish a meal you're thinking about the next meal or snack or treat. What it feels like to monitor every single bite that goes into your mouth, even every bit of sugar-free Jell-O. I have heard many stories, and I feel so grateful to my patients for being vulnerable and sharing them. I feel incredibly fortunate to have spent these years as a physician and, in a way, a confidant. And now I'd like to share their wisdom with you.

This book is for all of us: Those who have obesity. Those who love someone with obesity. Those who know someone with obesity or simply want to better understand health. Obesity is not a matter of choice or willpower but a chronic, complex disease rooted in biology. The chapters that follow trace what we now know about how the body regulates weight by defending its energy stores, why shame and blame only deepen the struggle, and why health—not appearance—is the real goal. There's been a breakthrough—a fundamental change in our understanding. The new medicines are transforming the treatment landscape. The science is moving so quickly that even doctors struggle to keep up, while patients are bombarded with mixed messages. We'll explore the most persistent myths. Losing weight does not mean you're "cured," food noise is real, medications do not work the same way for everyone, and while there can be side effects, as with any medicine, these are not inevitable or necessarily long-lasting. We discuss each one with a clearer picture of the science.

The field is changing unimaginably rapidly. With every new study, every new patient story, and every new medication, we are uncovering more about how biology drives behavior and how treatment can change lives. This book is about that science but also about the possibility it opens up—for my patients, and for you.

In these pages, or as you listen, I invite you to become curious and to set aside any preconceived notions about obesity: what it is, what causes it, and how to treat it. I invite you to open your mind to understanding obesity through the evolving knowledge of our biology and how your brain ensures that your body always has *enough*.

—ANIA M. JASTREBOFF, MD, PhD

1

Enough Shame and Blame

Obesity Is a Disease, Not a Choice

Oprah: If you've never had to struggle with your weight, I know it may be hard to understand the dread of seeing a certain number on the scale, a number that feels like defeat, proof that once again, the fat won, and you didn't. To buy clothes not based on what you like, but what will fit. And best cover you. What it feels like to be mad at yourself month after month and embarrassed year after year. To wonder how it's possible that I know how to do many worthy, life-affirming things and yet—no matter how disciplined I am, how strict I am with myself, how much I deny myself—I cannot control my weight.

How self-defeating it is to know that no matter how many times I said, "This is my last diet!" I couldn't keep that one promise to myself.

One of my strongest memories, what should have been one of the proudest moments for me, is veiled in embarrassment and shame. I was on full red carpet display and wanted to disappear. It was the 1992

Daytime Emmy Awards. I was anxious and nervous not for the reason you'd think—I didn't want to be there. I was the heaviest I'd ever been, 237 pounds, and in the weeks before the show, I couldn't find anything to wear. So, I'd had a custom suit made—a gold skirt and chocolate-brown jacket. I was so embarrassed to even go to the seamstress. Normally, during the fitting, I would say, "You can't measure me! You just have to look and take a guess." But this was a very public event, so I stood still, closed my eyes, and cringed, while they measured my bust, my waist, my hips. The designer did her best—a beautiful silk pencil skirt, a jacket with French cuffs in the same material—but I still felt so uncomfortable, so heavy, so exposed. I remember praying, "Please don't let them call my name. Please don't let me win, let it be Phil (Donahue) this time," because I couldn't bear the idea of getting up out of my seat, knowing everybody would be watching the back of me as I walked up each stair to the stage. Of course, they called my name, and I forced myself to smile and accept the award.

I left that ceremony and headed to a spa to try to jump-start myself to lose again.

I think now of the hours and hours and days and years of wasted time and energy I've devoted to losing and gaining weight, and how truly astonishing it is to learn, after all these years of blaming myself for the failure, that it is not and never was about willpower. That it's about your brain—and how your brain is going to fight to get you back to the weight that you were trying to lose. Understanding this has been profoundly liberating for me—and it offers all of us such an opportunity to release the shaming and blaming.

Oprah's stories are incredibly relatable and real, echoing what I hear daily from the patients I see in clinic and the participants enrolled at our trials at Y-Weight. Most people who come in seeking care have been unjustly, tragically shamed for having a disease. In turn, they criticize themselves. They chide themselves. They try and try and try to lose the weight. They continuously blame themselves when they fail, just as the world has blamed them.

My patients describe the feeling of being exiled to plus-size sections or stores failing to even carry their sizes. They describe the airlines that require them to buy two seats or necessitate an ask for a seat belt extension and then, like my patient Lynn, sitting through the entire flight stiff and rigid "like in a coffin" because she did not want to "take up too much space." My patients tell me about the constant barrage of ads that always find them—weight-loss supplements, herbs, patches, and creams— promising quick fixes. Other patients with less severe obesity tell me they feel uncomfortable. All the time. Because they have a disease. And the world has told them it's not a disease. The world has repeatedly told them that it's their fault—and this translates to many feeling that they are weak. That they are gluttonous. That they can't control themselves.

Meanwhile, their biology is telling them: I need a slice of deep-dish pizza. They might try to be satisfied with a veggie-packed salad with chipotle grilled chicken (maybe with a little fat-free ranch dressing?), but their biology says, "I'm starving! I need more energy! I need to store more fuel, more fat, just in case I run out!"

This is the disease of obesity. And quite honestly, if we were living during a famine, a time of scarcity, people with obesity would have an advantage. Their brains' pull to store more energy would better protect them against starvation. But in our modern world, in an

21

environment that encourages storing extra energy, there has been a shift in how much fat all of us store. In a way, we are all predisposed to store more fat. People who one hundred years ago would have been characterized as "normal" weight now are overweight. People who were genetically predisposed to be overweight now have obesity. For many people with obesity, food chatter can drown out all other thoughts. A litany of diets rob those with the disease of the time and attention they could spend going bowling or learning to play the guitar or to speak Mandarin.

While still not recognized and accepted by everyone, medical associations including the World Health Organization and the American Medical Association recognize it as a disease. But obesity is not a disease because various associations recognize it as a disease. Obesity is a disease because it is a medical condition with complex underlying biology that negatively impacts health. For now we can say that obesity is incited by our modern environment and occurs when our brain instructs our body to store more fat than it needs. This extra stored fat results in detrimental impacts on health.

The definition of obesity is still a contentious topic, and maybe this is part of the problem. And the limited definitions and descriptions we do have don't communicate how it feels to have the disease. Not everyone who gains weight has obesity. However, if you have it, you know it. You've tried 621 diets and none of them work. Or if they do work for a few months, then they stop working. Many think about food, food, food. Day and night. Morning and evening. You wake up sometimes and eat all the leftover turkey meat loaf from dinner, then sit in the kitchen and berate yourself. Or maybe you don't eat the turkey meat loaf. You resist. You throw it out. Then sit in the kitchen, wishing you hadn't. You wasted food. Your kids could have made meat loaf sandwiches. You can weigh 195 pounds or 495 pounds or 295 pounds. The number on the scale doesn't matter. Whatever you do or don't do . . . you never have enough.

And what does that not having enough and storing extra fat translate to in terms of our health? Well, what are the top two causes of death in the United States? Heart disease and cancer. Does obesity increase the risk for developing heart disease? It does. The lifetime risk for developing heart disease in people with obesity (without diabetes) is close to 50% in women and nearly 70% in men. That translates to one in two women, and two in three men. That risk goes up even further in the presence of diabetes, and nearly 90% of people with type 2 diabetes have obesity. What about cancer? Having obesity also increases your risk of developing certain types of cancers. At least thirteen types of cancers have been identified as being obesity-related, including postmenopausal breast cancer, colon cancer, endometrial cancer, pancreatic cancer, thyroid cancer, and the list goes on. In fact, there are more than two hundred obesity-related diseases and complications. So, let's imagine a world where we can safely and effectively treat obesity and, in so doing, potentially prevent, mitigate, or treat hundreds of downstream diseases, in effect saving lives.

We don't have to imagine such a world; we are living in that world. We have safe and effective treatments.

Now is a transformative time, an exhilarating time, a hopeful time. But as thrilling as this moment is, it's important to recognize what it truly means—and what it doesn't. These medications are not "magic" as some refer to them, nor do they erase the complex reality of obesity. They are tools that help us target the biology of the disease, but, as with many chronic diseases, they do not cure the disease. To understand just how redefining these medications are, we need to step back and look at obesity for what it really is: not a matter of choice or a failure of willpower but a chronic medical condition rooted in the body's own regulatory systems, which are responding to our current environment. This is the crucial shift—from blame and shame to science and treatment. Obesity is *not* a moral failing. It is not a choice. It's a disease with an underlying biology that causes harm, due not only to the physical burden but also to the weight of the world's judgment—judgment that people with obesity turn against themselves, beating themselves up long after the world and social media have gone to sleep.

Where Do Shame and Blame Begin?

Oprah shared with me that the seed for her feelings of shame began in her teens, well before she ever developed obesity. As she mentioned earlier, her childhood memories about food were positive. She also did not think about weight. It was in her late teenage years, while she was living with her father in Nashville, that her feelings began to change.

Oprah: I remember I had just gotten a scale, and my father said, "Oh, you don't have to worry about that. No need to weigh yourself. Because you gonna be big. No matter what you do, you're always going to be big. Have you seen your momma and your momma's sisters? You come from a history of big people. I once had your mother and her sisters in the back seat, and it was hard for me to drive off, because they weighed down the back of my Buick." I remember that moment and

I carried that with me through every marathon, through every *Vogue* cover, through every book, through every episode on weight. Somewhere in my subconscious was the voice saying: "You're gonna be big. You're gonna be big. Have you seen your aunts? Your mother?"

While her father did not have the experience of having obesity, he recognized the pattern (which had genetic underpinnings) in Oprah's maternal family. He couldn't have known that to his impressionable adolescent daughter his words would be a recurring message of self-blame and become part of her inner dialogue over the years, every time she gained weight. He simply stated what he had observed.

During the Oprah YouTube special with WeightWatchers, called *Making the Shift*, we heard many stories of the shame people carried with them over years. One young woman named Steph shared a story on the livestream that had happened decades before. "When I was in high school, I thought I looked so good in these jeans and [I wore them] to a dance," she said. "The next day, the pictures came out and a girl printed the picture [of me] out and made copies and put 'cow' all over it and put it in a hallway.... I didn't think anything was wrong before that, but now I started to envision myself as a cow walking through the halls. All I heard was 'moo' every time I would think about my body.... It's imprinted in my heart.... I thought the only way to solve it was eat the carrots and drink water.... I'm a Latina, and I have curves ... I was told that curves were not beautiful. I was told curves are considered 'fat' and you need to change it. I wanted to know what those hip bones and that neckline looked like on me.... To see that is something I always wanted as a teenager ... and never achieved." Such stories from our childhood or adolescence have profound impacts on our self-perception.

The Self-Hatred Voice

Amplifying what society or well-meaning friends or family say, there's no harsher critic than our inner voice. The soundtrack of self-blame can be louder, crueler, and more unrelenting than anything anyone else might say aloud. On that same livestream, Oprah was joined by actress Rebel Wilson. Oprah read a passage from Rebel's memoir that captured the cruelty of that inner voice: "I'm a proud female. I've used my weight to my advantage. On the other hand, I'm ashamed of my eating behaviors. I feel guilty. I feel unlovable. I emotionally eat. I overeat. I'm addicted to sugar. I know I'm carrying excess weight and eventually it could lead to serious disease. I know that my father died of a heart attack a few years earlier with complications due to diabetes. I know that I'm often in pain after a long day's work—my legs, my feet, my lower back. I know that at thirty-nine years old, I've trashed my body with junk food, I guess because deep down I think of myself as trash." Hearing her words read back to her, Rebel teared up. "It's like still quite raw . . . It makes me sad because . . . why did I think like that?" I remember that moment well—sitting there listening to those words, my heart sank, feeling her anguish. The room collectively sighed with sadness.

Self-blame is one of the most pernicious effects of shame. It convinces people that every struggle with weight is a moral failure. Self-blame manifests as that mean inner voice. "It's no one's fault but my own that I gained weight," the voice says. The guilt piles on. The cycle becomes self-reinforcing: Blame leads to shame, and shame leads to self-blame, which then fuels self-shame. And because the voice is internal, it often feels inescapable. Not all, but many of my patients with obesity share with me that they have this inner voice. It says, "I know I shouldn't eat the burger-fries-shake combo. That's bad for me. *I* must be bad. If I only eat the carrots, I'll be good." It's heartbreaking—and given what we know now about our biology, it's tragic that we think this about ourselves. But we created this society and an environment that fueled this.

My patient Alice began experiencing self-blame in childhood. Her well-intentioned mom put her on diets when she was in her early teens. Even before that, she had started to develop what she eventually called the "self-hatred voice." She vividly remembers when she was ten years old, sitting in the front yard with her legs bent, seeing the inside curvature of her leg and wanting it to be smaller. "This is the line where your muscle is, and on the inside is a curve. That's the fat and the extra skin. I thought, 'Oh, if I could just cut that off, then my leg would be perfect.' I had a pen, and I drew the line where I thought my legs should be and where the fat should be cut off. I just knew that I was larger than I wanted to be."

Alice lived in Vermont at the time, and her mother had a garden where she grew all sorts of vegetables—lettuce, carrots, cucumbers. "I just remember eating salad, so much salad!" Alice recalls. At thirteen, she sat at the table, thinking, "Here's a plate with three pieces of lettuce and a carrot," and wondering how she was going to get through basketball practice or soccer without passing out or blowing the game for her teammates.

A few years later, her mother put herself and Alice on a no-carb diet. "Atkins was kinda big," Alice says. Her father and two younger brothers were exempt; it was only for the girls of the family. Which basically meant Alice and her mother were still eating everything from the garden, except no turnips, because turnips had "too many carbs."

After three days, Alice revolted. She reached for some crackers in the cupboard: "Mom, I just ate an entire sleeve of saltines!" Hearing this, her mother was not upset with her. Alice shared, "She was desperate for carbs, too, and ate three saltines herself. And then dutifully returned to her no-carb diet."

At sixteen, Alice started tracking her weight for sports. The self-hatred voice in her mind began to be very specific and explicit. "The cupcake you just ate—what is the number of calories in it? What is the number of carbs?" She described that it wouldn't let up, not even for just one tiny-teeny bite. It was unrelenting.

Fast-forward more than thirty years, and by the time Alice was nearly fifty, she had tried every diet and workout program under the sun: forty-seven of them, to be exact. Atkins, keto, South Beach, the Zone, low carb, no carb, ultra-low fat, liquid only, Jillian Michaels, Jane Fonda, Suzanne Somers, full-body HIIT workouts, gym memberships, a YMCA weight coach, DietBet, StepBet, a Mediterranean diet, a vegetarian diet, the raw food diet, intermittent fasting. She'd even tried hypnosis. She had three teenagers, a fulfilling job in communications, and a loving boyfriend. She struggled with obesity despite spending much of her adult life tracking every morsel of food, eating mostly healthful meals, and exercising every day. She had successfully lost weight countless times. That wasn't the issue. The problem was that she always gained it back. She always blamed herself for having obesity. She did not know about the biology of obesity, yet.

The Perils of Self-Shame

There are other far-reaching consequences of societal blame and shame and self-blame and self-shame. Small things like parties that are skipped or more serious things like doctors' appointments that are never made, mammograms missed or never scheduled. I hear about this from my patients: The fear and worry that they will yet again be judged has often delayed them from making the phone call or walking through the door of the clinic—for months or sometimes years. Research studies confirm this; every aspect of our health care system, including health care providers, has condemned patients for decades. It's one of the main reasons I try to ensure that my study participants and clinic patients feel validated, welcomed, and accepted the moment they reach out or walk through the door to see me or any members of my research team.

Because of self-shame, some moments and some decisions can't be taken back, and may lead to lifelong regrets. Julius shared just such a story, in the context of his lifelong struggle with obesity. When he was a baby, his mother and father told his grandparents that they were going to the store—and then they never came back. Raised by his beneficent grandparents, Julius turned to food to cope with his parents' absence and being bullied and ostracized in his small town. He started overeating in secret: sneaking cookies and hiding food under the bed. He developed obesity at a young age: "I remember shopping at Huskies with my grandmother as a child," he said. He continued to gain weight in college and, during his freshman year, was diagnosed with diabetes by a school nurse. "I beat myself up, thinking, 'What is wrong with me? Why can't I stop eating?'" He thought, "I must be unlovable."

After the diagnosis of diabetes, Julius tried to lose weight in every way he could find. He tried different diets and attended Overeaters Anonymous 12-step meetings, weight-loss rehabs, and other programs. A family member even supported him through several of these, including for binge eating disorder that co-occurred with his obesity.

Throughout the years, he struggled, feeling depressed, and despite loving and missing his grandparents, he rarely returned to his hometown. The shame of having obesity, as he described it, "remained an albatross around my neck." Julius depicted himself as hiding and working to become invisible not only to the world but to those he loved most—his grandparents. He would visit rarely and only right after he had lost weight in a program.

"One day, I got a call from my family that my grandmother was dying," he said. "All I could think was 'I have to lose weight, because they're going to tease me and talk about me back home.'" His anxiety and fear set in, just thinking about being at the funeral: "People are going to think I'm still not good enough." Julius hesitated, trying to figure out how quickly he could lose five pounds. Two days after getting the call, he booked a flight home. The same day he was flying to see her, his grandmother passed away in the early morning hours before he arrived. "I was too late." He didn't have a chance to see her before she died. "I never forgave myself for that. In my mind and in that moment when I got the call, the pain of being teased and feelings of shame and embarrassment were far greater than anything else to me. The fear felt palpable, paralyzing, and real to me. And this is the woman who raised me and who I loved, right? That's what I've dealt with—a life of regrets, a life of shame, a life of missed opportunities, a life of pain, and a life of suffering. When society heaps shame on us, we turn against ourselves—and we hurt ourselves even more. And we miss so much of life."

A heartbreaking story mired in self-shame. When I first heard Julius share his story on a panel, I was so moved I instinctively reached out to hold his hand to support him as I listened.

The Battle Against Shame

Personal blame and shame take so much from people with obesity. Society's condemnation evolves into stigma and bias and unfair treatment. Starting in the late 1960s and early 1970s, movements and organizations began to form to fight for the rights of people living with obesity, to combat bias and stigma, and to promote self-acceptance and self-love. Because obesity is an externally visible disease, for decades the focus has been on appearance rather than on health. This is now shifting. It is beyond the expertise of this book to delve into this history, but it is important to highlight that no one should ever be blamed or shamed or face stigma for having a disease. From the health care lens, the cornerstone of compassionate care is empathy, respect, and nonjudgment, regardless of circumstances or whether or not a person is seeking treatment, just as it is for someone with any other condition that affects health and well-being. Whether it's diabetes, depression, or obesity, compassionate care and respecting patient autonomy is key.

Jill, a mother of five, who was a member of the audience at the *Making the Shift* YouTube special, spoke to the challenge of finding that same empathy and nonjudgment within herself. She wanted to make sure that her eight- and eleven-year-old daughters loved themselves. "I try to teach them that we love our bodies for what they can do for us. 'Cause we can go swimming! We can go to school!" she said. "But inside I really don't feel that way, and so it shows up in everything that I do every day. I don't want to go out with my friends because I don't want to be the biggest one there.... I haven't gone shopping in fifteen years because I just can't feel good about myself." When her daughter asked why she always wears black, she said it was her favorite color. "In reality, I hate wearing black," Jill admitted. "I'd much rather wear pink or other colors." She had been taught that black clothing was slimming.

Jill said she grew up in a world where one "had to be skinny to be happy." She struggled with this all her life, wearing black, standing in the back for photos, missing events and activities because of her obesity. "I don't want them to feel the shame that I've felt my entire life about my weight," she said about her daughters. As for herself? "I want to love my body for the five kids that it gave me, but inside it's really difficult."

Although Jill was trying so hard to have gratitude for her body, it was challenging for her to believe that we all are beautiful and glorious and that we come in every size, each of us with our own biology.

She's not alone. Oprah shared her thoughts on that same livestream:

Oprah: I so wanted to be like body positive advocates. I was trying, in my own way, to come to loving myself. I've done all the exercises and the meditations. I've been to India, and I sat with the gurus. I've done it all. But it's hard to love yourself when the rest of the world is constantly telling you that what you look like isn't good enough.

The Perniciousness of Shame and Blame

After the forty-seven diets failed her, Alice reached out to participate in one of our clinical trials at Y-Weight. The trial was one of a new medication, called tirzepatide, that was being developed for the treatment of obesity. What happened over the course of the next year and a half transformed her life and her health. She lost nearly half her body weight, her knees stopped hurting, she stopped counting every calorie, she stopped keeping a daily weight chart on her bathroom mirror, and in her own words, "I stopped being mean to myself." Before starting the medicine, she ate healthfully, tracked every morsel of food, exercised every day, and went to PTA meetings. After starting the medicine, she ate healthfully, tracked every morsel of food, exercised every day, and went to PTA meetings. The *only* difference was that with the medicine, she lost weight. Near the end of the trial, I asked her what this experience felt like. She captured the biology of obesity treatment with these new medications in one succinct sentence: "It's just as easy to lose weight as it ever was to gain weight." Finally, her brain felt that her body had enough. She felt a sense of ease. In fact, the origin of the word "disease" is "lack of ease." So treating the disease brought her ease. It wasn't until Alice took the medicine that she slowly began to understand and believe that biology was the real cause of her medical condition. Alice was living the biology. She knew that she was doing everything exactly the way she had done it before the medicine. And without the medicine, it was almost impossible for her to lose weight and maintain long-term weight loss. But with the medicine, she was able to lose the weight and keep it off. She began to understand that it wasn't her fault.

Or so I thought.

At the end of the trial with tirzepatide, Alice had to stop the medicine for a month and then come in for one more visit. Many studies require some time off the medicine before the final visit so that the participants' health can be assessed and safety can be ensured. Less than a week after that last study visit, she came back to see me not as a participant but now as my patient in clinic. "I've gained twelve pounds in four weeks," she said. She was near tears.

"It'll be okay," I said. "It's not your fault. It's biology. We'll try different medications to address the biology of your obesity."

Alice knew (intellectually) that usually after the medicine is stopped, most people start to gain back weight. It's the same as if someone stopped taking their insulin; their blood sugars would go up. But it's very different to know something on an intellectual level versus living it. She felt awful about gaining back weight, but she wasn't doing anything wrong. This was simply her obesity's biology fighting to gain back the weight she had lost with the medicine.

We had discussed all of this together before she stopped the medicine, but it's hard for someone who's lost weight with these new treatments to imagine what might happen without them. Alice told me later that it felt like she had finally gotten real help over the course of the nearly year-and-a-half-long trial, and then it was taken away. In Alice's case, without the medicine she would eat the portion size she had eaten while taking the medicine, but just a short time later, she would be hungry again. She couldn't stop herself from going back for seconds. She was relentlessly pulled to eat "all the pasta, so much pasta," she said. She would wake up in the middle of the night hungry.

So, even though we had talked about all of this ahead of time and even though I continued to convey to her that she was not at fault, it was still difficult for Alice not to blame herself. I couldn't put her back on tirzepatide; it wasn't available yet. So, to try to slow down the weight regain, we started another medicine—a very good one, but not as effective for Alice. Of the ninety pounds Alice had lost, she regained about half, and then her weight plateaued. We then added two more medications, to get her to a place where her health remained improved and she felt well.

About a year later, once tirzepatide became available to her, I sequentially transitioned Alice off the other three medications and switched her back to tirzepatide. She felt comfortable at her current weight (about seventy to seventy-five pounds down), where she has remained to this day.

Alice surprised me during a recent visit when she confessed that despite all those years we spoke about biology—and all those years she has lived with her biology both on and off medications— only now is she starting to truly internalize, understand, and embrace that it really is biology that determines her weight, not her willpower. Since she began taking tirzepatide, she knew it was working, targeting her obesity biology, but letting go of the idea that somehow she was in control and responsible for her weight was something altogether different.

That's how intractable the shame is, along with the belief that we are ultimately fully in control.

And it's also why it really matters how we talk about these medications. The words we use can suggest the false idea that they're just "weight-loss drugs." They're not. These are obesity medications. Medicines that target the biology underlying this chronic disease. Let's consider what obesity actually is—when the parts of the brain that manage energy stores start telling the body to hold on to more fat than it needs. These medications help recalibrate those signals so the body then wants to store less energy, less fat, helping to restore us to more health. That is why people who take the medicines not only lose weight but maintain weight loss.

Obesity is a chronic disease, not a choice. Treating obesity is a lifelong process. We now know that targeting the biology to recalibrate the set point treats the disease itself—and that this can also potentially prevent or treat hundreds of other obesity-related conditions. Taking obesity medications is not the "easy way out"; it is treating the biology of the disease.

Sometimes I am asked how it is that I don't blame people for having obesity. My answer is simple: Could I blame my father? I never thought it was his fault or choice. He just never quite felt full or satisfied with the amount others ate. He wanted seconds and that was his brain, his biology. At some point he crossed a threshold, he developed obesity, and his brain just wanted more; it was never *enough*.

At the time, we didn't understand the biology, and so blame filled the gap, but science has since confirmed that it wasn't his fault. Just as it wasn't Oprah's, Alice's, or Rebel's fault, or that of any one of my patients or participants or the millions of others who struggle with obesity. Obesity is a complex, chronic disease.

Oprah: I want to acknowledge that I have been a steadfast participant in the diet culture that contributed to some of this shame. Through the magazine, through the talk show for twenty-five years, through online channels—I've been a major contributor to it. I cannot tell you how many weight-loss shows and makeovers I have done. That famous wagon-of-fat moment on *The Oprah Winfrey Show* is one of my biggest regrets. It sent a message to the people watching that starving yourself with a liquid diet was a standard—that neither I nor anybody else could uphold. Maya Angelou always said, "When you know better, you do better." That's one of my favorite teachings from her, so the conversations online, on TV, and in this book are my effort to do better. Recognizing once and for all that obesity is not a moral failing, that it's a chronic, relapsing disease—that has been life-changing for me. I did not get the memo ten years ago, but now I know and I want to spread that information to as many people as I can. Whether you choose to start moving more, whether you want to eat differently, whether you want to change your lifestyle, whether you want to take the medications, or whether you choose to do absolutely nothing because you are satisfied exactly the way you are—that's up to you. Whatever your path, though, all I ask is that we stop the shaming of others' choices.

2

Chasing Enough

What Is Obesity? And Why Do I Have It?

I pause for thirty seconds and recenter before seeing my next patient. We have not met before; this is her first visit. I knock on the door, and I walk into the clean, spacious exam room at our new Center for Weight Management at Yale. Sitting on the exam chair is Carla. She's exquisitely put together in a beige pantsuit, a teal bag at her feet. According to her chart, she's forty-eight years old, five foot five (1.65 m), and 236 pounds (107 kg).

Also in her chart is her BMI, or body mass index, a calculated measurement that is weight (in kilograms) divided by height (in meters) squared. Carla's BMI is 39.3 kg/m², which is at the top of the range of class 2 obesity. The World Health Organization (WHO), defined the severity of obesity into three classes. Class 1 is defined as a BMI of 30 to 34.9 kg/m², class 2 is a BMI of 35 to 39.9 kg/m², and class 3, or severe obesity, is a BMI of 40 kg/m² or more. It's important to note that BMI was *not* designed as a diagnostic tool; it was designed to be a screening tool. The calculated parameter was initially created as a research instrument used to compare the amount of body fat relative to height across large numbers of people in studies. That way, hundreds of people could be quantitatively compared to hundreds of other people even though they all had different builds. BMI was never intended to be used for decision-making for individual patients, yet this is what has happened.

Health care providers currently commonly use BMI as a snapshot or a yardstick to screen for and diagnose obesity, owing to its low cost and simplicity, but its clinical use is not without flaws. At the individual level, the measurement does not account for the amount of fat (versus lean mass, including muscle), the distribution of fat (where it is located in our bodies), or the sex, age, race, or ethnicity of the adult. In fact, the predecessor to BMI was developed in the mid-nineteenth century by a Belgian statistician, astronomer, and polymath, Adolphe Quetelet, who concluded that weight increases at the square of one's height. He based his findings of "Quetelet's Index" on measuring Western Europeans in the 1800s. In 1972, Ancel Keys, an American physiologist, coined the term "BMI," validating the calculated index by analyzing height and weight data from nearly seventy-five hundred men from five countries (US students, executives, and railroad workers; rural Finns and Italians; Italian railroad workers; Japanese fishermen and farmers; and South African Bantu men). Insurance companies eventually started using BMI, whereas they had previously used "weight by height" tables accounting for sex and body frame, to determine "ideal" body weight, as they recognized that excess weight was a predictor of accelerated mortality by examining longevity data. So, BMI is not without flaws. We eagerly await the development of additional tools to help diagnose and characterize obesity. Obviously, my patient Carla is not a white European man. As I learn from our conversation that morning, she's a working mother of three who has a thriving law practice. She came to my office before work to talk to me about her weight.

Defining Obesity

Obesity is actually not a number, and I am guessing Carla did not make the journey to see me because her weight divided by the square of her height puts her at the top of the class 2 obesity category. She is also not here because the number on her bathroom scale reads 236 pounds, though this is an objective measure that relates to why she is here to see me. While these numbers may have varying degrees of meaning, my challenge during this visit is to understand how having obesity impacts her life and her health. She is here because she has obesity.

The WHO first recognized obesity as a disease in 1948 and currently defines obesity as "abnormal or excessive fat accumulation that presents a risk to health." Here the emphasis is primarily on "health" (and not a number) and this is an extremely important concept echoed throughout this book. Notice the definition doesn't distinguish what kind of health, be it mental, cardiometabolic, orthopedic, respiratory, or any others. It doesn't explain what degree of excessive fat constitutes obesity, address why there is abnormal or excessive fat, or make a judgment as to how the individual with this condition acquired the extra fat. It also doesn't refer to diet or why the person cannot lose the weight or keep the weight off.

I extend this definition, thinking of it slightly differently, and find it to be helpful both for me and for the patients I care for. As a physician specializing in the care of people with obesity, I consider that *obesity is a disease where the weight-controlling regions of the brain inappropriately instruct the body to store more fat than is healthy or needed.* This occurs in the setting of our obesogenic environment.

You'll note that the focus is on the biology (physiology) of the disease and includes the brain. This is key, as obesity is a neurometabolic disease. A more in-depth definition could be: Obesity is a chronic neurometabolic disease characterized by the storage of excess or abnormal fat that occurs when the brain inappropriately instructs the body to store more fat than is healthy or needed.

You'll also notice that nowhere in any of these definitions does the word "obese" appear. Many of us grew up saying and hearing things like: "Sally is obese" or "Tony is obese." Many of us might also remember referring to someone with alcohol use disorder as an alcoholic or someone with diabetes as a diabetic, but all of these terms are intentionally and actively being faded out of use, because they imply that the person is defined by their disease, not that a person has a disease. We need to make that same change in the setting of obesity and stop using the word "obese," moving to person-first language. The diseases someone may have—including obesity—are just one aspect of their lives and do not define who they are.

Whenever I meet a participant or a patient, I try to get a sense of what words they prefer to use with their disease. Do they use the words "weight" or "BMI"? Do they use the word "fat"? Are they already comfortable with the word "obesity"? While I respect whatever my patient's choice may be, I hope that within my lifetime we no longer use the word "obese." Wouldn't it be great if that word was removed from our vocabulary? Instead we all would say a person "with obesity" or an individual "has obesity."

Meeting Carla

"Thank you for coming in to see me," I say. It's her first appointment with me in the clinic. As mentioned earlier, my "day job," as the director of the Yale Obesity Research Center (Y-Weight), gives me the opportunity to meet with people who have obesity and are interested in participating in clinical trials of new obesity medications. Because these are new therapies—which are being investigated to assess their safety (adverse effects and side effects) and efficacy (ability to change weight and other health measures) so that the FDA has the information it needs to decide about approval for clinical use—participants need close monitoring in the research setting. This means that with my clinical research team, we have frequent visits—often monthly, more or less—with each participant, allowing us to spend substantial time together. In contrast, in the routine clinical setting, patients are seen every few months and for shorter appointments. This reflects the broader health care system's structure, which generally isn't designed to support frequent patient visits for chronic conditions. While that challenge extends beyond the scope of this discussion, it underscores how essential it is to establish trust and rapport with each new patient. My work is not just about medicine and science, it's about relationships, compassion, and care, and I want to lay a good foundation with my new patient, Carla.

The first thing I do is try to figure out how she is feeling this morning. Does she seem anxious to be here? Excited to meet me? Uncomfortable in a doctor's office? Hopeful? Ashamed? Empowered? All of the above at once? Sensing how a person feels helps me determine what to do and how to frame and phrase what I'm going to say to ensure it reaches my patient. My job is to help make Carla, and every other patient I meet, feel safe, heard, and validated—the opposite of judged.

She is sitting very still and very straight with her ankles formally crossed. Perhaps she is a bit nervous, but her steady gaze conveys to me that she's ready to talk about why she faced the frustrating Wednesday-morning traffic on I-95 to get to Yale.

"Thank you so much for seeing me," she says.

"Of course." I smile reassuringly, and I sit down to be at her eye level. "As we begin, I'd like to say that whatever we talk about, whatever you share with me, there is no judgment. You can say anything that comes to mind. I just want to hear about you from you. You are here because you would like my help, and I'll do what I can to help you." I pause and watch her face for any shifting emotions. "I usually begin by inviting new patients to share their weight journey with me. Tell me about your weight. When did you first become more conscious of your weight? Begin to gain weight? Lose weight and then gain it again, or have other medical or life struggles? What has worked and what has not worked for you? What have been your challenges and your successes? Please feel free to share anything you'd like."

As with all my new patients, I ask Carla these questions, and then I stop. I don't look at any screens, any of the patient's electronic medical records. I don't type on the keyboard. I've been told, though I don't realize it, that I mirror the body position of my patients. So maybe I cross my ankles and sit quietly too. I wait. I listen.

Most of the time, the patients' stories come fast and furious:

"Well, I gained a lot of weight with my second pregnancy with my son. And I said I would lose it straightaway. He's seventeen and I just never lost it. Instead, I gained forty more pounds."

or

"Well, I don't remember ever not being 'the chubby one.'"

or

"I remember my mom signing me up for WeightWatchers when I was fourteen."

or

"I started taking several medicines for my mood in my mid-twenties. They really helped my mood but I gained fifty pounds on these meds."

or

"I was always very active through high school—the baseball team, the basketball team, running cross-country. Even in college, I played pickup basketball and kept up my running. Then I broke my ankle skiing one winter break, and never really ran again. After that it seems like my metabolism just slowed down."

or

"Well, I just can't stop gaining weight. . . . I just can't."

The stories about weight are never the same. Neither are the happy stories in between the tales of frustration and disappointment—ones about the wonderful, fulfilling lives lived, lives that I want to know all about. My patients' jobs, their partners and pets. Their hobby as a watercolorist, their church choir or neighborhood bocce ball league. The childhoods that shaped them, whether full of poverty and struggle or wealth and ease. I focus on these details because I want to know who the person is, what the person loves about life, what they love about themselves, and what brings them happiness and joy. I want to know about that, and help them hold on to it themselves, despite the shame and blame that inevitably surfaces when they talk about their weight:

"I stopped eating in the cafeteria in the third grade. I didn't want anyone to see me eating my smooshed half PB and J sandwich or my chocolate chip cookies."

or

"Dining with colleagues, I would order a mixed green salad with a small piece of grilled salmon for my entrée. I'd intentionally leave half the fish, drink Diet Coke, skip dessert—except maybe just a single bite of Black Forest cake, because it was my childhood favorite—but usually I'd skip the dessert just so I wouldn't be judged by my dinner companions. All I could do, during the entire dinner, was think about how hungry I was while I watched my coworker, with judging eyes on me, devour a sixteen-ounce rib eye with a loaded baked potato, a bottle of wine, and a giant piece of Oreo cheesecake. After dinner, I'd race home, starving, and, out of view, eat my second dinner—cold roasted chicken leftovers and string cheese. It's not fair."

or

"Every day for breakfast I have the same plain Greek yogurt with berries. For lunch, canned tuna, cottage cheese, and an apple. And for dinner, a salad with grilled chicken. I work to get in about eight to nine thousand steps a day, but if I even look at dessert, I gain weight. I try so hard and am hungry all the time. I wake up in the middle of the night thinking about food. I have three teenage boys at home who I love dearly, and they all eat nonstop. The cupboards are crammed with their carby snack foods. I've started going to the grocery store early in the morning right when it opens, because I could no longer hide my embarrassment at the disapproving looks of other shoppers who see me and my overloaded basket full of foods the kids eat."

Self-blame may emerge in various ways throughout the stories:

"I promised myself I would lose those fifteen pounds, but instead I gained another sixty."

or

"I know I should have exercised more but, instead, I focused on my career."

or

"My mother told me I am better than this, and I believe her. I know I am . . . but still I keep failing."

Society has heaped on blame and shame for years. I often hear a recurring refrain: that while they realize it's not helpful to be mean to themselves, they're just not able to stop.

Carla is not different. "I hate my belly," she says. "No matter how much I work out, I can't lose it. And it's gotten so much worse with perimenopause. Even though I've been stuck consistently between 231 and 236 pounds, somehow I've had to go up two pants sizes in the last year. I get tired by three o'clock and the day's just beginning when I get home to the kids. It's all so frustrating. I don't know what else I can do."

She continues sharing the most intimate details about her struggles with weight, beating herself up for eating the tamales and coconut cake last weekend at her niece's quinceañera and lashing herself with negativity because she told her son—and promised herself—she'd walk fifteen thousand steps every day after her shoulder surgery, but she keeps coming up short.

Now Carla is crying, her mascara running down her cheeks. I feel my eyes well up. I'm trying not to cry too, but it's hard. I feel my patient's struggle and want to do all I can to help, to take away the pain, the blame, the shame. I hand Carla a box of tissues, taking one for myself just in case.

But I have the answer for her.

As soon as she has her Kleenex and is dabbing her face, I swoop in with . . . biology.

By biology I mean human physiology—in other words, how a body works. Biology that determines how, when, and why we make and store fat.

So, here's the truth—the truth for Carla and everyone else: Our bodies are hardwired to respond to environmental cues and factors like stress, flavors, seasons of the year, even the hour of the day. In terms of our inherent biology, there are traits that are handed down by our parents, grandparents, and great-grandparents over generations. I explain to Carla that our bodies are doing *exactly* what they were designed to do. Humans evolved to survive scarcity: bodies built to store energy, brains wired to seek calorie-dense food, muscles designed for constant movement. Many of us know this story— we're optimized for a world of famine and flight. The problem is, we now live in an opposite one. Today's landscape is what researchers call obesogenic: an environment that nudges us (if not hurls us) toward weight gain at every turn. Our bodies were never meant to exist in a world of ultra-processed foods, desk jobs, no respect for rest or sleep, endless screens and pings, and stressful commutes.

I share with Carla that our bodies are responding to confusing cues and signals from our environment, it's just that those signals have changed, and our biology is being tricked by the environment into thinking we do not have enough. This is what I want to make clear to all my patients: If you take a body that has evolved in one environment and put it in a dramatically different one, the consequences can be profound. I also want my patients to know and understand that some bodies may respond quite differently to these changes compared to other bodies—that there is an explanation for why they struggle with their weight, but their neighbor might not. Our brains control how much fat we store and they are great at their job, especially in an environment of uncertainty and scarcity. But in our current environment, which promotes obesity, there has been a shift in how much fat all of us store. In a way we are all predisposed to store more fat. People who were genetically predisposed to be "normal" weight are now overweight, and people who would have been overweight are now developing obesity. The entire weight (or fat storing) curve has shifted up for the population of the world. For most people there is not one gene that accounts for how much fat our bodies store, but rather a genetic predisposition to hold on to more or less fat.

Why Do We Have Fat?

Let's talk about what fat is, why we have it, and why, even though at first glance it may not feel like the case, fat is actually a wonderful "innovation" that allows us to live and function and survive as a species. Essentially, fat is a storable form of fuel, and it is our primary stored source of energy. If you want to learn more about the science, check out the Notes at the back of the book.

The term "fat" can be confusing because it can be used to describe the molecule that our body stores and burns as an energy source, but it can also refer to the tissue or organ where fat, the fuel, is stored (also known as adipose or adipose tissue). When you look at the nutritional information on a bag of chips or bottle of olive oil, "fat" is referring to fat as a fuel. The sixty-seven pounds of "fat" Oprah wheeled onstage in her red wagon was fat tissue. This tissue form of fat secretes important signals, such as hormones, that communicate to our brain the amount of energy stored as fat. In addition, it serves as a protective tissue providing cushioning, like cellular Bubble Wrap. Where it is not obvious in the book, I'll distinguish between fat the fuel and fat the tissue. Fat the fuel and fat the tissue are both good. It is only when there is excess fat the fuel either stored inside fat the tissue or overflowing into other organs not meant to store so much fuel that we start to get into trouble.

Our body uses energy all the time. And to make energy, we burn fuel. That means when we go on a bike ride, drive our kids to school, make dinner, do laundry, kiss our partner good night— even when we read, breathe, and sleep—we are burning fuel.

What are the sources of immediate fuel for us humans? Food. Fuel can be mashed potatoes, garlicky broccoli, enchiladas verdes, smoked salmon, a juicy peach, lentils, latkes. Food has three principal components, called macronutrients. The three are: protein, fat, and carbohydrates.

We all know what protein is: steak, fish, chicken, tofu, tempeh. Fat-rich foods include butter, oils, avocado, and nuts. Carbohydrates are foods like fruits, vegetables, bagels, pasta, bread, and sugary sodas. Carbs are mainly sugars, although importantly, not all carbs are sweet-tasting. There are also other carbs, such as fiber, that are very important but not used for energy.

The food we eat is most often a combination of these three macronutrients. We need to consume all three—protein, fat, and carbohydrates—because they enable us to do four things: build, burn, store, and dump. We build muscle and other important body components (bone, skin, hair, nails, even enzymes) with protein; we burn fat and sugar to make energy to do things such as walking; we store fat so we can burn it later; and we eliminate the byproducts that we can't use—also known as pee and poop. Here, we're just going to focus on how our body burns and stores fuels like fat and sugar.

The two principal sources of fuel that we burn are carbohydrates (sugars) and fat. We need energy all the time, but we can't eat *all* the time—if we did, we wouldn't have any time to work, do laundry, mow the lawn, read a book in the park, or anything else. Our bodies need to have a way to store that fuel, so we can use it at a later time. That storage is crucial and is part of our evolution. Back in the cave days, there was no Instacart, and there were no supermarkets. The only fast food was creatures that we humans were too slow to catch. We didn't always have immediate access to food, and so we had to use parts of our bodies as personal pantries to save fuel for later.

What kind of fuel does our body want the most? Depends on what part of the body is using it. Our brains *love* sugar—more than all other fuels. By weight, the brain makes up 2% of our body, yet it hoards about a quarter of all the glucose for itself! The brain cannot directly use fat as an energy source and so it mainly uses glucose. Sugar has an extremely important, and sometimes exclusive, energy-supplying role in our bodies. In addition to our brains rapidly chewing through glucose by thinking, dreaming, and remembering, some muscle fiber types also use sugar exclusively as a fuel. Escaping from a raging tiger, running for a touchdown, or chasing the ice-cream truck can burn through our sugar supplies pretty quickly. Sugar is super important for survival, winning football games, and, ironically, getting more sugar. If our brains and muscles depend on sugar so much, then why do we store energy as fat? One simple explanation may be that storing all our energy as sugar would take up a massive amount of space in our body, compared to storing it as fat. This would be very impractical.

Our body's sugar economy is run on glucose as the main carbohydrate currency. In the grocery store, we can buy pure forms of sugar as powder, crystals, and cubes, but our bodies can't use it or store it in these forms. For sugar to be used, it must first be dissolved into our body's water. Once it enters our bloodstream, it can then circulate to and between different organs, some of which (especially liver and muscle) have the capacity to store sugar. Under normal conditions, glucose in the blood is very dilute. That is, there is only a little more than four grams of sugar in our blood at any one time (about the same amount as a teaspoon of table sugar, a single strawberry-flavored Starburst candy, or four to five McDonald's french fries). Too much sugar in the blood is called diabetes mellitus, where the too-high glucose spills into the urine, literally giving us "passing through sweet" (which is the translation of the words "diabetes mellitus"). If all our energy was from sugar, we might burn through five hundred to a thousand grams (approximately one to two pounds) of sugar a day. That would be up to twenty-five hundred grams (five pounds) a day for Michael Phelps during Olympic training!

But remember, we don't have cubes of sugar in our blood. The most concentrated form of sugar in our body is called glycogen— and it's composed exclusively of glucose. Because of its chemical nature, for every gram of sugar, the glycogen grabs and holds on to three to four grams of water. Think of it this way: Have you ever overestimated the amount of dry pasta it takes to make macaroni and cheese? One cup of dry pasta will grow into three cups of soggy, overcooked elbows, because the starches in the pasta love to hold on to water. Now let's imagine if you were to pour a cup of extra-virgin olive oil into a pot of water. If you were to decant the oil back off the top of the water, no matter how much you mixed or stirred, you would get back about the same amount of oil that you started with. Water and oil do not mix. That's because fat hates water (fat is considered *hydrophobic*, which literally means "fear of water"). Basically, sugars (e.g., glucose, glycogen, linguini, bread, potatoes, rice) take up four to five times as much space and weight as fat (e.g., canola oil, sesame oil, butter, lard) to store. Our bodies are not big enough. Humans would need to be four to five times larger (maybe like a dromedary) to store all our energy as carbohydrates instead of fat! But actually, we would be even larger, because there's more to the story.

Fat can store more energy than sugar.

Every one gram of sugar contains about 4 kilocalories of energy, while one gram of fat contains about 9 kilocalories of energy. So, by weight there is about twice as much life-sustaining energy available in butter compared to granular sugar. Uh-oh, now we are going to have to revise our size metaphor to include both the amount of water weight added to dry sugar as well as lower "energy density" (how much energy can be stored for a given mass). That means we would need as much as ten times the space and weight if we carried our energy as sugar instead of fat. We would need to be the size of a Bengal tiger. Not practical (but it would be pretty cool to be able to run up to forty miles per hour and have popcorn-smelling pee!).

So, on a per-weight basis, fat is ten times more efficient than sugar at storing energy. Smart body! As I mentioned earlier, all this is to say: *Fat is actually a good thing!* And storing fat is a good thing. Without the ability to store fat as fuel, we would die.

I can't say that at this point in the appointment patients share my enthusiasm for the role fat plays in our bodies, but I can see them beginning to realize that it's much more complicated than they—or anyone around them—had originally thought. The goal is just to know that like all things in life, nothing is all good or all bad, and that having the ability to store energy as fat is actually a very good thing.

So let's answer Carla's question: Why does she have obesity? Obesity is essentially your brain thinking that you are not storing enough energy even though your body has more than enough. Your body, and more specifically your brain, wants you to store more fuel—which, as we've just learned, means more fat—and so it's working overtime to figure out how to make sure you do that. Even if you are not using a lot of fat at the moment, the body wants to store some for later, to ensure you have enough energy to live. Like a Boy Scout: Always be prepared! This brain process is not conscious. We don't think to ourselves, "I better store ten more grams of fat so that I have 90 kilocalories on reserve and have enough energy to vacuum the house later." It's not about willpower either. It's about our brain subconsciously receiving signals from our body and determining what our body needs and then enacting a strategy to get it.

The Fat Pantry

In a hurricane or zombie apocalypse, you might run downstairs to your basement "nuclear bomb shelter" to grab a tin of Spam, extra-crunchy peanut butter, or that can of Hormel chili that you shoved down there during COVID. In the same way, it's great to have fat in storage for when you need it.

In fact, there are times we need to store a lot of fat. For example, we need fat as we enter into the developmental stage of puberty to fuel growing taller and hormonal changes. We need extra energy while pregnant to keep the baby growing, and afterward to provide the baby with breast milk. The human body's fastest period of growth is during the first year of life. Babies need a lot of fat, as they're using a large amount of energy to wriggle and crawl, along with needing fat as insulation to stay warm and to be protected from falls. Even more, they need a ton of energy from fat to mature and grow their baby brains. These are clear examples of times in life when accumulating extra adipose (fat) tissue is essential.

I can practically see the thought bubble above my patient Carla's head. "But what happens if you're not a baby or a teenager or a pregnant mother-to-be? What if you're a busy lawyer who is in perimenopause and keeps having to buy larger-sized slacks?"

Even if we're not in one of these stages of life, we still need to do all the things we do in our everyday lives—and so we need to store energy as fat so that we don't need to eat continuously. Fat actually does many other things besides storing energy. Fat the tissue produces special hormones called adipokines, it protects organs, and it plays a role in immune function. Fat also acts as a thermal insulator. When it is snowy outside, it helps keep us warm, just like the insulation in a house. That's why your thin great-grandma is always cold—she has less insulation. Fat is also a cushion. When you hit your elbow, it hurts a lot more than when you bump your thigh. As my colleague Dr. Donna Ryan says, "Fat is not the enemy." It is when we overflow from healthy to unhealthy storage depots that we get into trouble.

I explain to Carla that for some reason—and right now, we don't know exactly why—her brain is convinced she needs to store more energy (as fat) than her body actually needs. This excess fat can cause problems. Having a body with a lot of fat stored inside it means some of the fat (the fuel) may overflow and spill out of fat (the tissue) into other organs. And that makes it more difficult for our organs to do their main jobs, because now they're also moonlighting as fat-storage facilities (e.g., fatty liver). Additionally, our organs have to work harder. It takes more effort for our hearts to pump blood to all our organs and tissue, for our kidneys to filter fluids, because larger bodies need more blood volume to deliver oxygen and nutrients to all parts of the larger body. It takes more effort for our pancreas to make enough insulin so we can use all that glucose (in the setting of more fat our bodies make more insulin—because the insulin does not work as well anymore). Over time, our organs get tired from this extra work. Our legs and muscles also need to work harder to run a 5K—or just to take us up the stairs—if they're bearing more weight. Other issues can arise when we store too much fat over too long a period of time, including various health problems. The consequences of this can sometimes be seen immediately, and sometimes they take time to be noticed. For example, when we store extra fat in our liver, muscles, and pancreas, it's more likely that we'll develop diabetes.

Oprah: I weighed 210 pounds in my thirties. I was very overweight, but my blood pressure was still 110 over 70. The doctor was always amazed. But as I got older, that started to change. It went up, and my blood sugar numbers also started to elevate. Before I joined Weight-Watchers in 2015, I had been diagnosed as having prediabetes. Losing weight on that program helped me stabilize my blood pressure and blood sugar numbers, but in my sixties, I started having pain in my joints. By 2021, I'd become more and more debilitated—to the point where it was hard to walk down even a few steps. I needed a double-knee replacement—that's two surgeries, three months apart, with weeks of intense rehab. When I came home after the first surgery, I literally could not lift my leg. I couldn't even lift my heel off the bed! I vowed if I was ever able to get up again and walk around that I would take advantage of being able to be fully in my body. I'm grateful to be able to move in this world without that pain, but I believe carrying that extra weight over the years contributed to needing those new knees. And science tells us that that extra weight made me predisposed to eventually developing prediabetes.

During this first visit, I ask Carla why she is seeking treatment. She shares with me that she has worked hard to build all she has in her life—her family, her career, her home. But no matter what she achieves, she always feels like she has to work a little harder to "prove my worth" because she lives in a larger body. She tells me that she started her own law practice after she had been passed over for promotions that others got—and attributed it to being "seen as less" because of her larger body. She has started to feel pain in her back and hips even though nothing about her walking and exercise routine has changed since having her third son fifteen years ago. "Is it just age? Maybe it's weight?" she thinks. Multiple health care providers have told her to lose weight. But how? She puts just as much effort and dedication into "eating right, and getting those steps in" as she does with her work and family. She feels like in this one part of her life she has failed. She feels like her weight is holding her back. Even worse, she feels like *she* is holding herself back.

I share with Carla that it's our job to help recalibrate that biology so her brain does not think it needs to store quite so much fat. She nods and crinkles up the tissue in her hand, her eyes no longer teary. Like with many of my patients, I know that it will take time for Carla to embrace and understand that it's not her fault. Together we begin to make a plan.

There is an arc to every new patient visit . . . anxiety, hope, excitement, perhaps some wariness felt by the patient. Creating a safe space, listening, sharing the biology (*a lot* of biology). Lifting blame, starting to let go of shame, discussing treatment options, setting expectations, and beginning the journey . . . together. It is among the most rewarding work I do.

3

The Enough Point

How Your Brain Defends Your Body Fat

Oprah: I still have the check I wrote to my first diet doctor—Baltimore, 1977, I was twenty-three years old, 148 pounds, a size 8, and I thought I was fat. The doctor put me on a 1,200-calorie regimen, and in less than two weeks I had lost ten pounds (there's nothing like the first time . . .). Two months later, I'd regained twelve. That was the beginning of the cycle of discontent, the struggle with my body. With myself. In 1988, a little over ten years later, the number on the scale was 211, so I did a liquid fast. For four solid months, I didn't eat a single morsel of food. Well, that's not exactly true. I was at a hotel and broke down and ordered a burger with avocado. I remember running around opening all the windows to air out the burger smell before Stedman got back from golf. But that was the only solid food I had. Yes, I lost sixty-seven pounds—the "red wagon" pounds—but as I mentioned, by 1992, I'd gained all that weight back, and more, so I booked myself into yet another weight-loss spa. Only this time, I met Bob Greene. With his help, I lost seventy pounds. I yo-yoed over the next decade or so, but in 2004, I was probably the fittest I'd ever been. I ran my first and only marathon (26.2 miles). Just five years later, in 2009, I'd gained forty pounds back. When I got a call to ask if I would like to join WeightWatchers, I thought, "It's so bad that WeightWatchers is calling me?!" But because of that prediabetes diagnosis, I decided to try it. I joined the board in 2015 and started following that program. When I add up all those major weight losses—oh, wait, let's not forget the twenty pounds for the *Vogue* cover—it's over two hundred pounds. That's a lot of weight. It would take *three* wagons to show just how much that is. Yet it doesn't even count the five or ten or twenty pounds I'd lose and gain over and over and over between those monthslong efforts. Which must be hundreds more.

Losing that much weight is no small feat. That took an immense amount of effort, dedication, determination, and time.

So, when Oprah lost weight repeatedly, by diligently tracking her food consumption (every single morsel, from morning cereal to after-dinner Tofutti Cuties), limiting portion sizes, eating very healthfully, and exercising, her body seemed to initially respond. The pounds melted off, she was sleeping better, she was feeling better, and her clothes fit differently . . . But then something shifted. Oprah was doing all the same things she had done to lose weight, but now all those same things were no longer working. It got harder to continue losing weight—or even to keep the weight off. Over time, it felt as if her own body was fighting her, really *trying* to gain back the weight. And she did gain it back. Every. Single. Time.

What gives? Why did she yo-yo? With all the available resources and the mental fortitude of a summiting Mount Everest mountaineer, Oprah was understandably frustrated. But actually, we now know what was happening.

When we lose weight (or more specifically, when we lose some fat stores), our energy expenditure goes down (that is, how much energy our bodies exert) and our appetite goes up (that includes hunger, cravings, desire to eat). Let's focus on the energy expenditure first. As we lose weight, we become more efficient at using the food we eat, and in turn we need less food to do the same things we did before. The more weight we lose, the more efficient our bodies become, but only up to a point. Eventually, the efficiency is as good as it can get, because we still need to think, move, breathe, and have beating hearts. (Our body won't let us decrease our energy expenditure indefinitely until we perish.) Likewise, if we intentionally overeat and start to exceed our needed fat stores, then our body becomes less and less efficient and uses more energy to do the same things we did before. We burn more. Again only up to a point, then we start to put on weight.

To investigate this, Drs. Rudy Leibel, Michael Rosenbaum, and Jules Hirsch of The Rockefeller University conducted an elegantly designed study. In this study they intentionally put participants in a very controlled research setting (with their approval!) and oversaw every morsel of food they ate, noted every bit of movement they made, and measured how much they peed and pooped, how much oxygen they consumed, and how much carbon dioxide they exhaled, over weeks to months.

First the researchers studied the participants at their normal baseline weight, which they had all stably maintained for a while, and then, by controlling the amount of food they ate, the researchers had participants intentionally either lose 10% of their body weight (by limiting their caloric intake with liquid meal replacement) or gain 10% of their body weight (by compulsorily increasing the calories consumed to about 5,000–8,000 kcal per day). The researchers found that those who lost weight became more efficient (burned less energy) and those who gained weight became less efficient (burned more energy) by similar amounts regardless of whether they had obesity to start with. So this study taught us that our body adjusts how much energy it burns based on whether it perceives us to be above or below where our fat stores were at baseline. Basically, our bodies want to get us back to where we started.

Another study, this one conducted nearly forty years ago, demonstrated that mice that were overfed, underfed, or fed at will subsequently gained, lost, or maintained their weight, respectively. When all the mice were allowed to then eat as much chow as they wanted, the mice that had previously been overfed or underfed all reverted back to their original weight. In humans this has been shown with studies of various diets. After a period of maintaining weight loss in the setting of a diet, and thus some degree of caloric restriction, over time people gain back most, if not all, of the weight. Taken together, this suggests that our brains have a memory of how much fat our body wants to store at any one time. Our bodies go back to whatever the brain perceives to be the appropriate or optimal fat stores. So, when people lose weight by caloric restriction, the amount of fat stores their brains want them to maintain does not change—it is not decreased, and therefore they are subsequently pulled right back up to their baseline weight or, more specifically, their baseline fat stores. In the same way, when someone is trying to gain weight (let's say an actor for a specific role) by overconsumption of calories, the amount of fat stores their brain wants them to maintain does not increase during that brief period of time. So, once they are done with the acting role and go back to their previous food intake, they are pulled back down to their starting weight or, more specifically, where they were at baseline in terms of their fat stores.

In the scientific world, we call this phenomenon the "body fat set point" or "the defended fat mass." These terms capture the idea that our body tightly regulates energy stores. "Defended fat mass" is a way of describing how different parts of the brain work together with signals from our body to hold on to a certain level of fat, essentially defending and protecting the body's energy stores for survival.

A helpful way to think of this is that we have an internal "thermostat" that measures how much fat we are storing, and it can change how much we eat and how much energy we burn to keep us at a certain "body fat set point." For simplicity, let's call the "body fat set point" the Enough Point.

The Enough Point describes the brain's intention. The brain is working to maintain a state of equilibrium relative to the amount of energy it thinks the body should store. It's working to ensure we have the fuel and energy it predicts we will need. It's trying to protect us in the best way it knows how. But remember, our environment has recently changed to be obesogenic. This environment confuses our brain into thinking there is not enough fat in our bodies. Our biology was designed to survive times of scarcity when there wasn't enough food, or the food supply was inconsistent. And the food that was available was very different than it is now; it was unprocessed: meats, fruits, nuts, and vegetables. At the time, humans were also constantly moving, migrating, hunting, eventually planting crops and doing every chore by hand. Now, our Enough Point keeps getting pushed upward by our modern environment. Our brain's weight control system thinks that too much is not enough. It's calling the shots, and yet we feel as if it's all our fault for not controlling our weight.

Feedback Loops and You

Feedback loops are a way that our organs and tissues communicate with our brain and then the brain changes our behavior and metabolism to make sure we stay internally stable. The scientific term for this is "homeostasis." One example of a short-term feedback loop is when it's chilly and the nerves in our skin send signals to our brains that we are cold. Our brain then tells our body to shiver to help maintain our temperature in a stable, healthy place (around 98.6°F/37°C). When it's hot outside, the nerves send a different signal to our brain. We sweat, and the water evaporating from our skin cools us off. We are not consciously controlling our sweating or shivering. Likewise, we don't blame ourselves when we have these responses. If we did not have these feedback loops, we'd freeze (hypothermia) or overheat (hyperthermia) and die. These are drastic examples, but there are innumerable feedback processes going on all the time in our bodies, and they are essential to our well-being. The Enough Point is one of them.

The Thermostat and the Brain's Enough Point

For this part, it may be helpful to refer to the figure (in Appendix, page 246) as you read or listen along.

The feedback loops used to defend our bodies' fat mass may seem very abstract and not relatable. But what if we think about an example from our daily lives: a house's thermostat. Imagine the thermostat is set to a certain temperature, a set point—let's say 70°F (21°C). What happens in the middle of summer, when it's hot out? The house starts to warm up and the thermostat—set to "auto"—senses the increase in temperature via electrical signals in a thermometer and turns on the air conditioner.

The thermostat is part of a feedback loop that acts as the temperature-regulating system of the house, monitoring the temperature and responding to changes automatically. When the house gets warmer (say 71°F) and is above the set point (70°F), the AC turns on to cool things back down. In this case, the cool air comes from vents and lowers the room temperature, and then the thermostat "senses" the temperature change and turns the AC off. As the sun continues to heat the room, the cycle starts again. The hotter it is outside, the more often the AC has to run to keep up. On the flip side, when it's cold outside and the house cools down (say to 69°F), the thermostat detects the drop and turns on the heater, bringing the temperature back up to the 70°F set point. So, whether it's heating or cooling, the thermostat keeps trying to bring the temperature back to your comfort zone, responding to whatever the environment throws at it. Lovely—everything is stable and comfy.

Think of your body's fat-regulating system in a similar way. Instead of a single thermometer and AC/heater unit working behind the scenes, your brain uses several different regulatory systems in the subconscious mind to monitor and control your body's energy stores. This internal feedback system decides how much fat your body wants to store. If you lose weight and drop below the Enough Point, your body reacts: It burns less fuel and ramps up your appetite (your hunger increases, you want to eat more, you may crave foods that are especially high in calories). All of this happens subconsciously, manifesting consciously in some people as hunger, craving, food noise, and the like, thanks to hormone signals sent to your brain. Just as the thermostat strives to keep the house at 70°F, your body works to keep fat stores at its preferred level. But if the system is confused by being placed in a challenging environment (like our current obesogenic environment), the feedback loops can get mixed up. Individual differences in genetics and life circumstances, including social determinants of health, can make some people more vulnerable to these disruptions. Depending on where and how people live, their access to and quality of food will vary. All of this alters where each person's Enough Point is set—and why it looks different from one individual, or one community, to another. On a population level, our collective Enough Point has increased. Meaning that one hundred years ago, people who would have been normal or overweight in this environment are storing extra fat and now have obesity. And people who would have had obesity may now have more severe obesity. Everyone's Enough Point has shifted up to some degree in our obesogenic environment.

Let's see how this kind of disruption plays out in our thermostat example. On a hot, sunny August day you decide to bake your Granny Em's famous apple pie because your brother, niece, and nephew are visiting. Now, for some reason unbeknownst to you, the thermostat regulating the temperature of the entire house was installed right next to the stove in the kitchen. Poor planning, because as you bake, the thermostat senses all that extra heat and mistakenly believes the whole house is that warm. To fix what it thinks is a problem, the thermostat starts blasting AC throughout the house, cooling rooms that aren't actually hot—just because the thermostat is getting spurious readings from its overheated environment in the kitchen. We'll use this scenario, where the mismatch that occurs when the kitchen is comfortably at the thermostat-set temperature but the rest of the house is cold, as a metaphor for obesity (where the brain is at the Enough Point but the body is carrying too much fat).

Other things can throw the thermostat off too. For instance, as you've been baking, the kitchen has become quite a mess, so you close the door, which blocks air from moving to the rest of the house, keeping more of the heat in the kitchen and the cool everywhere else. Out of habit, you light a cinnamon-scented candle and set it right below the thermostat, making that spot even warmer (oops). The mid-afternoon sun beams directly onto the thermostat as well.

The thermostat gets all these "hot" signals—from the oven, candle, and sunlight—so it keeps turning on the AC, thinking it needs to cool down the whole house. But as the AC keeps the temperature near where the thermostat is set, the rest of the house gets colder and colder. Eventually, you notice that your family looks a bit uncomfortable, rubbing their arms to stay warm in the living room.

Similarly, your body has its own "thermostat" to regulate body fat at its Enough Point. In this house metaphor, the kitchen represents your brain, and the thermostat is the part of the brain that monitors and regulates fat storage levels. When your brain thinks your body fat stores are low, it turns on its own version of the furnace: You get hungrier and seek out more food, and your body becomes more efficient at storing and holding on to energy. Ideally, the brain system would keep everything balanced as long as all the signals could be delivered and interpreted correctly. Obesity happens when the brain gets confused by the environment, so that it thinks the body has too little energy rather than too much. Instead of turning on the "AC" it instead turns on the heat, and consequently, your body holds on to more energy as fat. It's not that the thermometer is broken, but if something blocks or confuses these signals—like the kitchen door being closed—the feedback loop gets impaired. The brain might think everything is fine, while the rest of the body keeps accumulating excess fat, leading to an imbalance that's hard to bring back into balance.

Whether it's the body's fat or house's temperature that is being maintained, regulation depends on both internal factors (like genetics—the location of the thermostat) and external factors (like food, stress, sleep, physical activity—the oven, the candle, the sunlight). Just like the thermostat gets mixed signals, our bodies, and specifically our brains, are constantly handling confusing cues from our environment—like artificial flavors, preservatives, sweeteners, and ultra-processed foods. And it's not just about food. Our lives are filled with stress and disruptions our brains may perceive as signals that we're in a chronically stressful or dangerous situation, one where we better save our resources (i.e., fat) for the potential bad times ahead. Stress is coursing through our lives and our bodies. We get laid off. Our retirement savings collapse. Our child is struggling with school. Our smartphones are pinging us with a continuous barrage of inputs. This world disrupts our internal clocks, and sleep goes out the window. Modern life throws off our internal rhythms, while making physical activity less necessary—after all, we no longer have to chase down our dinner. And back to food. We can have relatively inexpensive, highly palatable, ultra-processed food delivered directly to our doorsteps, and at portion sizes three times what our bodies were designed to need. Our brains and bodies juggle all these factors, trying to keep us balanced, even when the signals don't make sense.

Of course, obesity differs from an HVAC system; for one, it's a chronic disease. It's like the thermostat has been miscalibrated so it thinks the temperature is 60°F when it is actually 70°F. It could also be that the setting has been increased inappropriately. Trying to reset the Enough Point with exercise, diet, clean eating, or willpower doesn't seem to work as easily as blowing out the candle, turning off the oven, or opening the kitchen door. It is as if once the Enough Point is pushed up by all these influences, we cannot return it to the initial intended "factory setting" on our own. The scientific community doesn't yet fully understand this in biologic terms, which is why we need more research to understand the mechanism underlying obesity. What we do know is that obesity isn't one-size-fits-all. It's a complex condition caused by many factors, and each person's situation and biology are unique. Unless a patient's condition is due to a very rare genetic issue, we usually can't pinpoint exactly where in the feedback system things went awry.

All that said, we have an incredible, beautiful, robust system to help us survive. Frankly, it is remarkable that it works as well as it does in the world we currently live in. It makes total sense that our brains are responding to the craziness all around them—our bodies are reacting to the environment that they are in. When our brain circuits, the ones designed to regulate weight, think our bodies are starving despite sufficient fat stores, our brains will ensure that our bodies perform two tasks extremely well: conserving energy and taking in more energy. We've already discussed the first task and that is to reduce the overall amount of work the body does as a way to conserve energy, so burning less energy to do the same amount of work (the fancy term for that is "increased metabolic efficiency"). The second task our weight-regulating brain circuits excel at is making someone want to take in more energy—eat more. So now let's turn our attention to this second task.

In a pivotal study conducted by Drs. Priya Sumithran, Joseph Proietto, and other scientists, participants with overweight or obesity were placed on a calorie-restricted diet for ten weeks. The participants lost weight, but what happened with their hormones was even more interesting. The levels of hormones such as insulin (the hormone that enables us to use and store glucose) and leptin (the hormone released from our fat cells that communicates the amount of body fat stores to the brain) went down, whereas the amount of ghrelin (the hormone that peaks right before mealtime and signals "I'm hungry!") went up. Accordingly, participant-reported hunger levels also increased. A year later many of these hormonal changes persisted even after the onset of weight regain. This study demonstrated that as we lose weight, our bodies' hormones respond in a way that promotes more food intake. So, as we lose more and more weight, our bodies fight back, releasing every signal that they can, to make sure we replenish energy stores. Collectively, we call these changes "metabolic adaptation." It's something Oprah is very familiar with:

Oprah: After my knee surgery, I was determined to use my body differently and take advantage of my ability to walk. So I started with a quarter mile of walking. Then a half mile. Then a mile. Always limiting myself to one meal a day. One meal plus working out helped me maintain my weight in the weeks after my surgery and during physical therapy. As I said earlier, I even lost some weight. I was feeling really good about myself: "I can keep it off," I thought. "I can do it, I can do it, I can do it." But it started to come back on, and I couldn't figure out why. Of course I blamed myself. I thought, "I'm not being strenuous enough in my exercise, okay?" Mind you, I was walking three and a half to four miles a day, but I upped my mileage. I needed five to six miles a day to keep it off. I'm now eating dinner by four o'clock, because it takes me five hours to digest my food. I don't know what it takes for other people, but if I eat at four o'clock, by nine o'clock, when it's time to go to bed, I sleep easier. But I'm gaining weight. So now I have to cut down my one meal: a small piece of protein, a couple of vegetables, a small piece of bread. I began to realize, "I'm walking six miles a day! I cannot give the whole day to walking and I can't eat less!" I knew if you reduced your intake and you increased your exercise that weight would come off. But I forgot that it's usually only for a period of time. As Dr. Ania says, the harder I tried, the harder my body fought back.

Simply put, Oprah's Enough Point—her "normal" defended amount of fat—was higher than the weight she was carrying with six miles of hiking and 4 p.m. dinners. So, the fat-mass-controlling regions of her brain told her body to be more efficient and burn less energy, while her hormones told her to eat more.

Oprah: Based on what I've learned about the Enough Point, my body wants to be 211 pounds. No matter what I do, my body is always trying to get back to 211 pounds. Before I pulled out the wagon of fat, I weighed 211 pounds. Before I committed to WeightWatchers, I weighed 211 pounds. Before I started training for my first marathon, I weighed 211 pounds. Before my knee surgeries, I weighed 211 pounds. My body is always trying to get to 211 pounds.

Classic metabolic adaptation. Oprah's body wants her to carry energy stores that land her weight at 211 pounds. Our bodies work incredibly hard to try to pull us back to that Enough Point. That is also one reason why I always ask patients what their highest-ever weight was during the course of their lives (not including pregnancy). It gives me a sense of where their bodies may be pulled up to, and although it's not always the highest weight, it at least provides a range. The Enough Point is very powerful, built for survival. If someone is intentionally living below their Enough Point, their brain and biology keep signaling: "Not enough. Not enough."

Understanding Metabolic Adaptation (Sort Of)

So, let's break this down. As we talked about earlier:

> fat = energy
> energy = ability to function
> ability to function = survival

How do our bodies know how much fat, or energy, to store—in other words, where to set the Enough Point? Scientists don't know the details quite yet. Neurobiologists and biochemical physiologists have been working for decades to try to find the answers. We know a lot more than we did even thirty years ago about how the body communicates to the brain about energy storage levels, and how the brain processes these signals to regulate energy expenditure and food intake. However, we still don't know exactly how the body decides how much energy to store as fat, and why that changes in different stages of our lives. We do think that the regulatory system is greatly impacted by the obesogenic environment. One study that demonstrated this point was led by Dr. Kevin Hall while at the NIH. He gave twenty people an ultra-processed food diet (e.g., hamburgers, fries) for two weeks, and during a separate time the same group of people were given an unprocessed food diet (e.g., fish, salad, whole grains) for two weeks. The participants were served the same number of calories during each diet and were allowed to eat as much or as little as they wanted of the food that was offered to them.

Very different things happened with each of the two diets. During the two weeks of unprocessed food, the participants *lost* on average about two pounds, while during the ultra-processed food diet the same participants *gained* on average about two pounds. What accounted for the difference? When the same participants were offered the ultra-processed food diet, they consumed more calories, about 500 more calories per day than with the unprocessed food diet. Additionally, it appears that the participants ate their food more quickly during the ultra-processed food weeks compared to the unprocessed food weeks. So the same group of people responded very differently to the two different diets. This study is a clear example of how people can be impacted by even a short-term change in the environment, in this case diet quality, which affected the amount of food consumed and resulted in weight change.

At present, close to 60% of our food environment is composed of processed foods. Not all of these foods are ultra-processed foods; some include more healthful processed foods like whole grain breads, roasted nuts, plain unsweetened yogurt—but they are all processed. All that to say, in our current world, it is not possible for pretty much any of us to live on whole foods alone (apples, avocados, berries, broccoli . . .). But what we can do is try to eat as much of those whole foods and other healthful foods as is feasible and as a society work toward as healthy a food environment as possible to help prevent obesity.

As with many diseases of the brain, there is much more we need to learn and understand. And obesity is even more complex, as it not only involves the brain and body but also communication between the two, so it is a neurometabolic endocrine disease. What does this mean? "Neuro" means having to do with the nervous system, or specifically the brain. "Endocrine" means having to do with hormones. "Metabolic" refers to the chemical process by which the body turns nutrients into fuel (for use or storage). So, obesity is a neurometabolic endocrine disease as it encompasses all of these. Let's delve a bit more into the complexity of this disease and our impressive regulatory system.

Here's an illustrative example. The USDA recommends an average adult consume about 2,200 calories per day, which works out to just over 800,000 calories per year. But the average American consumes more than 3,800 calories per day, or a remarkable 1,387,000 calories per year! Where do the nearly 600,000 extra calories go? Those excess calories don't seem to get stored as the anticipated amount of extra pounds (see Notes for more details). For many people, their body weight stays relatively stable over time, with gains of one to two pounds per year (that's the average weight gain of the population), which is much, much less than what would be expected from more than a half million extra calories consumed every year. That is a remarkable degree of control over body energy stores and therefore body fat. Go, brain, go!

To be able to regulate our body fat stores (and, by proxy, weight), we must first have a way to sense how much fuel our body is actually storing. That is, how do the body fat–regulating parts of the brain keep track of how much energy we have stored as fat?

One of the first clues to uncovering the signals that tell the brain how much fat our bodies store in adipose tissue (fat tissue) was the discovery of a hormone called leptin, mentioned earlier in this chapter. It is released from fat cells and communicates with the fat-controlling neurons in specific regions of the brain. We must also have a way to sense when we last ate (hormones are the signals that communicate this in large part) and how much and what we ate, so that our bodies know what is about to enter our blood circulation for immediate use or storage. Likewise, we need to predict the next time we will be able to eat (this requires executive functions, stress hormones, knowing the seasons, etc.) and how much work we must do (hunkering down for the winter, building a cabin, preparing for a triathlon). There are a lot of things to keep track of, in order to be able to judge just the right amount of fat to store. So, regulation of energy stores is complicated, and we must have many contingency plans and be able to make changes on the fly. Remember, even in our summer-day AC example, when we were working with just one input (temperature), one target (thermostat setting), and one output (AC on vs. off), we saw there were many ways for the control system to fail, even when working as designed. It is no wonder we are just scratching at the surface of understanding the biology of energy regulation and obesity.

We know that even though our regulation mechanisms excel at making sure we have sufficient energy stores to survive and thrive, storing too much fat is not good for our health, especially long-term. Beyond the impacts of obesity itself, we may also develop obesity-related diseases or complications. There's diabetes, heart disease, and certain types of cancer—colorectal cancer, endometrial cancer, pancreatic cancer, and multiple myeloma are just a few of the cancers linked to obesity. All told, there are over two hundred obesity-related diseases.

What "Weight-Loss Diets" Teach Us

Let's pause here for a moment and talk about what we've learned about the Enough Point from certain popular diets, by hearing about another patient. Lydia, a young, determined entrepreneur in her early thirties, was committed to improving her health and wanted to lose about fifty pounds. She came in to see me for the first time in the middle of winter, when Connecticut's snowy, cold weather had thwarted her running routine. She had just moved up to Connecticut from North Carolina, and without her regular high level of physical activity to prevent weight gain, the pounds had started to creep back on. Her back started aching and she no longer fit into her favorite running pants, and she hated that.

In our initial conversation, she mentioned that she had tried what she called "a keto diet" several times in her twenties and that she always lost fifteen pounds right off the bat. Then she plateaued—no more weight loss. The moment she even looked at a corn muffin or smelled an everything bagel, she gained it all back. More recently, she'd tried the diet again, and got stuck again, just as she had in the past.

In response to her story, we went on a little tangent talking about what "going keto" means. These diets are very high in fat and very low in carbohydrates, with adequate protein. The main macronutrient in the keto diet is fat. Now, you'll remember the importance of carbohydrates to replenish our glycogen stores. When we limit carbohydrates, the body starts to run low on glycogen, *including all the water bound up in it.* The reason Lydia initially lost weight rapidly (and then her weight loss plateaued after losing fifteen pounds) was that she had deleted her glycogen stores and there was very little glycogen in her body to hold on to water. Much of the weight can initially come off quickly (and, to Lydia's dismay, go back on equally quickly), because a lot of that initial weight loss is actually from dehydration. So, the rapid weight-loss phenomenon known as the "keto flush" is appropriately named because you are literally flushing weight down the toilet as extra pee.

Now, it turns out Lydia wasn't on a true keto diet. She was on a high-protein, low-carb diet, something closer to the South Beach Diet. She wasn't consuming *only* fat—she was actually eating quite a bit of protein—but the effect was similar: She had little sugar in her body, and without the carbs, the water flowed out. (Think lots of trips to the bathroom.) Indeed, while some of her weight loss was fat—as some of the fat is converted to ketones, and likely the diet involved some calorie restriction—much of the initial weight loss was water. And once the water was gone in those first few fifteen or so pounds, the fat burn went much, much slower. So slow, in fact, she thought the diet wasn't working.

Lydia's experience is a common one. Her body had an Enough Point set at a higher weight than her conscious mind wanted. She attributed the quick "success" resulting from a change in her diet as proof that weight loss is about willpower. But we now know better. We've seen metabolic adaptation is powerful and very difficult, perhaps near impossible, to beat. Can some people lose a significant amount of weight with diet and exercise alone and maintain it for a significant period of time? Yes. Is that rare? Yes. There are always exceptions and as humans we want to believe that we are those exceptions.

So just as for Carla, why Lydia's Enough Point was set above what was optimal for her health, the medical field does not yet understand. There are many theories about this, but the general agreement is that there are factors in our current environment that promote holding on to that extra fat and developing obesity; many people, perhaps the majority, are susceptible.

Beyond that consensus, heated discussions occur around what those environmental factors may be and how they impact on a molecular level what the brain may have initially perceived as "normal" and why this changes. It's not a surprise that there's disagreement as we still have much to learn. These days, many people are comfortable accepting our bodies' feedback loops in terms of temperature regulation—telling us to shiver when we're too cold or sweat when we're too hot—but that's because this theory has been challenged and adjusted over centuries. The body fat set point model was proposed in the 1950s, and while we've made great progress, there are many things we still don't know. How exactly does our body determine how much energy it wants to store? How much is this determined by genes and by what mechanism? What are the controlling inputs that affect the body fat set point aside from factors that include but are not limited to food, sleep, stress, physical activity, and weight-gain-promoting medications (many medications have weight gain as a side effect)? Are there things we haven't identified or don't have sufficient research to understand well as yet (say, the bugs that live in our guts, maybe microplastics, endocrine disrupters in our food and water)? Does it matter if these "stressors" occur during pregnancy, fetal development, puberty, adulthood, or menopause?

Other questions are equally bedeviling: The body regulates many other things, such as immunity and red cell mass, so why does it allow for this degree of extra storage of energy or fat? If the body can set plenty of other regulated limits—for things such as minerals, electrolytes, water—why is it that the limit is so much broader for fat storage? Why can we gain so much, even if it harms us?

But then we remember conditions like high blood pressure, where somehow the body has become confused and believes that a higher blood pressure is normal or good. That's similar to obesity, right? In the long run, the brain is acting against the body's best interest; such a complex issue to unravel.

In the meantime, we'll continue to discover more about our bodies' weight-regulating mechanisms and about the Enough Point. Researchers around the world are investigating these mechanisms now (if you're interested, please participate in studies or donate time or resources, and have patience and empathy for the science teams studying and working to better understand obesity). We have much to learn—and we will. Ten years from now, the contents of this chapter will likely be quite different.

Let's revisit my patient Carla at her first appointment: The idea of an Enough Point makes a lot of intuitive sense to her. She is nodding her head and starting to look back up at me. She definitely relates to the concept of her Enough Point being set too high. She's experienced the pull back up to higher weights many times. She is fully engaged, listening and sharing. We continue our discussion of metabolic adaptation to understand that while our bodies are becoming more efficient at using the energy we have, they are also putting food front and center in our minds, making sure that we seek it out. Constantly. Relentlessly.

4

Holding Your Breath

The Overwhelming Food Noise
You Can't Outthink

Let's do a little experiment. I'd like to invite you to hold your
breath. Start holding your breath right now as you read this page.
Get ready, get set, go! Hold your breath. Hold it. Keep holding it
as you read to the bottom of this page, and all of the next page,
and the next. Keep holding as you start the next chapter. Then
hold it until the end of the book.

Actually, just keep holding your breath for the rest of your
life.

If you intentionally held your breath, you may have noticed
it was easy at first, but became progressively harder. If you made
it to thirty seconds, perhaps all you could think about was taking
the next breath. Sixty seconds and the entirety of your brain was
screaming at you to breathe. Your body wants you to live.

That's what trying to control your weight through caloric restriction indefinitely is like. Monitoring and limiting every dollop of whipped sweet potato or bite of sourdough biscuit that passes through your lips for the rest of your life is like me asking you to hold your breath always and forever.

This analogy surprises people who have always heard weight management is about calories in and calories out. In part, they're startled because that in-out story had made sense: You start to eat less, and the numbers on the scale tick down. It's simple math. But as we've learned, the math is anything but simple.

Think about consciously planning and executing every breath of your life. You would not be able to sleep. In parallel, if you actually had the job of regulating exactly how much fuel or energy you were responsible for storing, you'd be crunching numbers every second of your life. There's addition and subtraction, to be sure, but so many more inputs go into this calculation. How much do I need to eat—in kilocalories? How much am I burning—in kilocalories? How efficient are my mitochondria right now? How old am I (and, by the way, how old are my mitochondria)? What biological sex am I? What am I doing at this moment? Am I doing it quickly, slowly, how intensely?

Let's say you are walking up the stairs. How much body weight are you carrying up the stairs? How heavy are the groceries in your arms? How high is your heart rate? Your heart is responsible for pumping blood and oxygen to your legs so that your muscles get energy to climb. It's also pumping blood to your liver so it can do its work. See? Suddenly we're way, way past adding and subtracting what we ate for lunch and what we burned at the gym. We're into some kind of biological calculus that our subconscious brains, with constant, continuous input from our bodies, do for us faster than any TI-85 scientific calculator. Thank you, brain!

I explain this complex real-time math to my patients because I want to underscore that thinking we can control our weight with calorie restriction (our metaphorical breath-holding) is just not possible long-term if you have obesity.

My colleague Ted Kyle shared another way to look at this concept that underscores this point. Imagine what it feels like to be out of breath—not by choice, but by necessity—whether from running after one of our grandchildren or pressing up a tough hill on a bike ride or struggling through an asthma episode during allergy season. We breathe heavily because our bodies want and need more oxygen, not because we are breathing incorrectly. "If you have asthma, we don't instruct you to 'breathe normally'; instead, we treat the asthma," said Ted. "When we treat shortness of breath, we address the physiologic problem, not the breathing behavior." He's right. We need to and should treat the underlying, neurometabolic biology of obesity.

Let's look at this another way that often resonates with my patients. We accept in countless other conditions that biology sets the terms, not willpower. For example, if we have diabetes, we don't think that we can concentrate really hard and *make* our blood sugars get to—and stay in—a "normal" range. Or if we have high blood pressure, we don't think that meditating will make our blood pressure normal as fast as we can say "om." Or if we're taking a statin medication for high cholesterol—we don't think that never eating a french fry again is the way to go. Even after eliminating a lot of fats from their diet, some people still have high cholesterol. We wouldn't expect those folks to throw out their medication, would we? We accept without question that we need medical help to make sure these diseases are controlled.

And yet, when it comes to obesity, despite all the work health care providers and researchers have done to get the message out about the biological principles and despite decades of research showing otherwise, we cling to the idea that we should be able to overcome biology by sheer force of will—and then blame ourselves when we can't.

This idea that somehow we can and should overcome our biology is such a corrosive and long-standing belief—undermining so many people's sense of self-confidence and self-worth—and I've thought about why this may be so insidious. Perhaps weight *feels* different, because we eat every day—multiple times a day—so we think we have autonomy over what and how much we consume. We feel responsible for every chocolate chip, every sweet cherry, every crumb at the bottom of a Funyuns bag that we put in our mouths. But, in large part, biology is in control.

Oprah: I feel like I've been controlled by potatoes for forty years. Any kind of fried potato, baked potato, scalloped potato–oh my, oh my. Potato chips? Forget it. I love salty and crunchy. I cannot keep a bag in my house. I remember traveling one day, and I opened a five-ounce bag of crinkle-cut black pepper potato chips and I counted out ten chips. And I ate the ten. I savored each and every one. And then I. Put. The. Bag. Away. When I told that story to a private WeightWatchers group, I joked: "Of all the accomplishments that I've made in the world, all the red carpets, and the awards and those things that I've done–the fact that I could close the bag and not take another chip? It's major for me." Again, I was *kidding*, but the fact is, resisting the urge to eat the rest of the bag—heck, not opening another bag—that had always felt impossible. I can think of so many other times, no matter how much I knew, no matter how hard I tried . . . I just could not make myself stop.

Meet the Messengers

So, if our conscious mind is not in the driver's seat, determining how much we want to eat, what we want to eat, and how much we store from those meals, then how does this happen? While we don't have all the answers yet, we know our bodies are very efficient at using the energy we have. But how do our bodies do this? Through carefully crafted, intricate communication systems between our bodies and our brains.

The three main messenger types in these systems are hormones, neurotransmitters, and nutrients. Yes, nutrients, like glucose, are not only fuel; they are also messenger signals. They inform neurons in the brain of minute-to-minute changes in the amount of immediate-use fuel, and they act across the whole body. Neurotransmitters, like dopamine or serotonin, operate on a millisecond time frame and mostly act locally. They are important in the immediate response to meals and help us experience many significant things such as reward or pleasure from that delicious piece of creamy dark chocolate or from listening to our favorite song. Hormones are the key messengers in the obesity story because they are important in helping to determine both the time and scale of a meal and the food consumed. They are also the longer-term regulators of how our bodies manage our Enough Point, and so that's why we're going to focus on hormones.

Getting Hormonal

Hormones get many pieces of information from organs and tissues, such as how much energy they are storing, and then tell our brains exactly what is going on in our bodies. Obviously, there are all sorts of hormones—just ask your teenager how they are feeling, and then ask again in an hour to get a sense of fluctuating estrogen or testosterone levels—but the sex hormones of puberty are different from the hormones that communicate about our fat stores.

Since you are reading this book, you are likely familiar with several of these hormones already. One that is getting a lot of headlines is GLP-1. Media coverage refers to the new obesity medications as "GLP-1s," but they are *not* actually GLP-1s. This is a misnomer and sometimes leads to confusion. GLP-1 is a hormone made and released in your body. Its full name is glucagon-like peptide-1 (it's fun saying that quickly five times in a lecture hall). It was discovered because its secretion from the gut is stimulated when we eat food. So, it is what we call a nutrient-stimulated hormone or a NuSH. Later we found out that GLP-1 is also released directly in our brains when we eat food. The GLP-1-based or, more inclusively, the NuSH-based medications are modified versions of this and other hormones that have been designed by incredibly bright chemists.

GLP-1 has a cousin that was actually discovered a few years before GLP-1. This hormone is named glucose-dependent insulinotropic polypeptide—so we call her GIP. GIP secretion from gut cells is also stimulated when we eat, so GIP is also a NuSH.

Other NuSHs include hormones like amylin, glucagon, and

polypeptide YY (PYY), as these are also secreted when we eat. Medications are being developed that are modified versions of these other NuSH hormones as well; you will see them in doctors' offices in several years. Chapter 10 delves into innovations in the pipeline and the newer NuSH-based medications to come.

Other hormones, such as leptin or adiponectin, are secreted from our fat cells—leptin in proportion to the quantity of fat cells we have, and adiponectin inversely to the amount of fat we have—and these hormones communicate longer-term signals to our brain. Since leptin is secreted in proportion to the amount of fat we have, this makes it a good signal from our body to communicate to the brain how much body fat is presently being stored.

Here's how hormones can play out in real life. Let's imagine a patient who is at a stable weight. The leptin-sensing regions of the brain register that her fat mass is on target. If she eats a meal, her GLP-1, GIP, and other hormone levels go up, and communicate with various regions of the brain that sense these hormones. These regions are often referred to as satiety centers, but it is more complex than that: There are also reward-motivation regions and decision-making regions of the brain, as well as a vital control center for survival called the hindbrain (and all these parts of the brain talk to each other!). These regions coordinate to do a calculation on the fly (somehow—with that brain TI-85 calculator) that then communicates the size and energy content of the meal and helps to let her know when to stop eating to keep her body fat levels, and thus leptin levels, relatively constant. This is the fine-tuned feedback strategy to help balance her food intake with the amount of fat she has. A reminder: None of this is conscious.

Now let's say she has decided to try to lose weight again, like the many times she has before. As her fat depots get smaller, they secrete less leptin. The leptin-interpreting part of her brain says, "Hey, your energy stores have decreased. We've got to do something about that because my 'sensors' are reading that you don't have enough body fat to get us through the winter!" Meanwhile, my patient's "I don't want to get diabetes" and "I wanna look great in this dress" part of the brain says, "Sorry, I disagree." This is where the lines are drawn and the battle begins.

After a few weeks, she has lost 5% of her body weight (that's ten pounds for someone who weighs two hundred pounds at baseline). When she eats smaller meals, her gut still releases the GLP-1 and GIP hormones, but the satiety regions and other regions of the brain sense the smaller amount of fat (via longer-term leptin signaling) and say, "Nope, we're not happy yet! Time to go back for seconds! We're worried that since you are eating much less, there may not be enough food around for the weeks ahead, and we must get prepared to make it through the famine." That there is no famine, has been no famine, is unlikely to be a famine in this patient's little cul-de-sac, does not matter in the least.

Being extremely strong-willed and able to push through the discomfort, at least for a few months, my patient decides that despite these hunger signals, she is done with dinner. "Perfectly satisfied with the portion," she tells herself. That night in bed, though, the leptin keeps pestering her about not having enough fat supplies to survive the upcoming challenge. Again, in the morning when she wakes, her brain is still having the same conversation. In fact, most of the time, she gets signals that she needs more, that what she's currently storing is not enough. And if she were to keep her weight at 5% below where she started, even after a year, the leptin-sensing regions would relentlessly keep pushing her to eat more. That's right, a year later, she'll still be fighting her brain trying to raise her body fat stores to the prior Enough Point.

Let's say this patient really wants to lose 10% of her weight for health reasons (that's twenty pounds for someone who weighs two hundred pounds at baseline). The same internal conversations would be going on, but they would get louder and louder throughout a greater majority of the day and night. The weight-controlling regions of the brain become increasingly frustrated. All of this discussion between her body and brain results in hormonal signaling—making her want to increase energy intake, perhaps by increasing cravings for energy-dense foods—because her body thinks it is starving. So, she's not only craving healthy apples, fiber-full oranges, and potassium-rich bananas, but also Texas BBQ Brisket–flavored Pringles potato chips ("fat and salt, crunch, yum!") and Ben & Jerry's Cherry Garcia ice cream ("fat and sugar, creamy, super yum!"). The hormones also tell her to keep eating. Say she made a well-portioned dinner. These hormones cause her to want to eat seconds or thirds, or dig into the Tupperware full of leftovers after everyone's gone to bed. These hormones are mighty. They have the strength and power of the signals telling you to breathe when you are holding your breath.

Even if she marches out of the kitchen or away from the table, her subconscious mind will keep thinking about food, like a nagging itch that needs to be scratched. All of this is very familiar to those living at a weight (more specifically, fat energy stores) below where their brain thinks it should be, living below their Enough Point.

That Very Noisy Food Noise

How does living below our Enough Point manifest consciously? It appears as "food noise," which is a symptom of obesity experienced by many people. Food noise ensures that a body gets the fuel it needs and wants to store (erring, as always, on the side of extra, just in case).

Many of us may think about food throughout the day, but for those with obesity living below their Enough Point, food noise is different. Food noise—which is defined as intrusive, persistent, and disruptive thoughts of food—is distinct from the sensation of being hungry before a meal or the craving we get after catching a whiff of freshly baked chocolate chip cookies straight from the oven. The latter two examples are sensations that are critical for our survival. If our brains did not have a hunger center, we would not have any appetite and we would not survive as a species. If we did not have reward-motivation regions of the brain, we would not experience cravings and have the desire to eat highly palatable foods that could give us that boost of energy we need to be prepared to run away from a lion or bear.

Food noise is different. It's a constant inner voice that just won't stop chattering on (and on and on) about food. Here's a hypothetical example that might give you a glimpse of what my patients describe.

Imagine this is your life: Monday you start your day with a Greek yogurt with blueberries and a splash of honey. You go to work and have a juicy Fuji apple for a mid-morning snack. You're working on a report that has a 5 p.m. deadline, but you just can't seem to focus—you keep thinking about lunch. You packed it the night before and it's sitting in the work fridge, waiting for you. You always try to resist eating until noon, but you cave at 11:47 a.m., just thirteen minutes earlier than you had planned—but you were feeling so hungry that you just could not hold out. You eat a huge green salad with tuna, dressing on the side. You sit back down with a cup of tea to finish the report, but fifteen minutes later, you still feel like you haven't had enough. You're distracted. "Focus," you tell yourself. Then count down the minutes until your planned after-noon snack—a baggie of almonds—but a colleague has brought in brownies, home-baked, from scratch, and asks if you'd like one. Yes—actually, no, drat! You're not supposed to eat those. But they are sitting there in the shared kitchen; even at your desk, you can smell the chocolatey goodness . . . You can't stop thinking about those brownies. You walk to the water cooler, have a glass of water, hoping this will quell the craving. No such luck. Your mind is now relentlessly preoccupied with the brownies. You resist them and their fudgy gooeyness . . . until 3 p.m. You make yourself a cup of decaf coffee, carefully cut a teensy-eensy piece of brownie, and go back to your desk. You savor each tiny bite of that small piece. You finish your report in the nick of time, then you go back for another teensy-eensy piece, which you eat over the sink, brush the crumbs off your blouse just in case anyone notices, and make your way home. You made it through the day. Barely.

You get home, and your second workday begins as you care for your family and their needs. Your husband is driving the kids to baseball practice, so you run to the store and then prepare a healthful dinner—salmon with lemon, arugula salad with sun-dried cherries and balsamic vinaigrette, and wild rice pilaf (wow, the epitome of healthy right out of a magazine). The kids eat some of the salad but want pasta, so you make them that as well. You make sure to drink water before and during dinner so that you stay well hydrated and take care of your kidneys.

Then the dishes are done, and you're all set until tomorrow morning's breakfast—your carefully planned-out egg-white-and-red-pepper omelet. But as you walk past the kitchen, something is gnawing at you. You remember your kids' Milano cookies in the pantry. "No, don't eat the cookies!" your prefrontal cortex, the decision-making part of the brain, says. "You resisted the brownies at work, except for those two little nibbles, you don't need a store-made cookie . . ." Then the thought sneaks in: "But those cookies are so yummy, with that butter cookie crunch and smooth dark chocolate." You think about the delicious, nutritious dinner you just ate. "Maybe one cookie is okay," you tell yourself. "Didn't the dietitian say you should not restrict foods altogether?" You take a bite of that scrumptious double-dark-chocolate cookie—it tastes so good. You tell yourself to stop after that one cookie, but then somehow you find yourself eating another cookie, and then another . . . There goes the rest of the bag. Oops!

You tell yourself, "No problem, tomorrow is another day. I'll add fifteen minutes to my walk and be all set." You make tomorrow's lunches for yourself and the kids, fending off thoughts of the ice cream in the fridge, and go to bed, feeling like you did "okay" but "should" have done better. You dread stepping on the scale the next morning. You fall asleep thinking about those rich, fudgy homemade brownies at work, and wondering if there will be any left tomorrow.

Where Does Food Noise Come From?

Many people with obesity or who are overweight are trying to live below their Enough Point (aka their body fat set point), and that can make food noise constant. In other words, no matter what the executive parts of our brain are telling us about our weight and our need to lose weight, food noise will come in like an insidious nag. For many people with obesity, food noise is unrelenting. That's why, over the long term, the executive regions of the brain don't stand a chance against the onslaught of minute-to-minute hormone signals that are howling for attention. The feedback loops (from chapter 3) are incredibly powerful, wired for survival, and not in our conscious control.

So why did food noise come up for discussion only when highly effective obesity medications became available? Why didn't we talk about it before? Well, sometimes we don't know something exists until it's no longer there. Oprah did not know that she was living in a cacophony of food noise until she experienced the peaceful silence. It was only after people with obesity shared that these thoughts were now quiet in the setting of the medications that we began to understand that food noise is a symptom of obesity and living below the Enough Point. The obesity medications are targeting obesity biology and quieting the food noise by recalibrating (lowering) the Enough Point.

People with overweight or obesity assumed that food noise was a normal part of existence, of being human—and it is, if you are living below your Enough Point.

Oprah: The single biggest surprise of taking the medication was waking up and *not* thinking about the very first thing I wanted to eat . . . or the healthier thing I should have wanted . . . or the bargain I could make with myself so I could eat the first thing . . . or maybe if I went with the healthier option for breakfast, the snack I'd reward myself with for being "good" . . . then the thoughts of how many hours before I could justify "snack time" . . . The endless noise and negotiations had always been there, rattling around in my brain, for so long that I'd just gotten used to them. The endless conversations with myself, no matter how draining they were. All felt normal. But after the medication, what I now know as food noise went away. I couldn't believe it! All those years, I thought the people who never had to diet were just using their willpower. I thought every single person was resisting temptation every single minute of the day. I thought they were just stronger than I was. Actually, I knew they were. They had to be. After all, they were thin, and I was not. But now I realize y'all weren't even *thinking* about food! It's not that you had the willpower; it's that you weren't thinking about your next meal. You weren't obsessing over what to eat. You weren't talking yourself out of what you were about to eat or what you absolutely could not eat. I remember years ago on *The Oprah Show* talking to a group of models—Christie Brinkley, Cheryl Tiegs, Beverly Johnson—about what they ate and hearing their concern about the size of their thighs. I thought, "Honey, I could tell you a thing or two about thighs!" I told them about the time I went on the Atkins diet and removed every single carbohydrate from my house. There was nothing in my refrigerator. There was nothing to eat, except hot dog buns in the back of my freezer. One night, I was so craving carbs, I took the deep frost off them, thawed them out in the oven, poured syrup on them, and ate them all, because I was so desperate. People who don't have the disease of obesity just don't think about food the way I and others do.

Now that food noise has been identified as a symptom of obesity and living below your Enough Point, researchers and clinicians are working to try to understand it better. There is even a Food Noise Questionnaire that was recently developed and is beginning to be used in studies.

Subconscious Grazing (aka "Who Ate All the Chips?")

Of course, for all the food noise that you wish would stop, there's another, much quieter phenomenon around food that can be hard to navigate. Take this example: It's been a hard week at work, but you are proud of yourself for a key project you completed, and ahead of time! And the fact that your kids made it to all their activities this week without a hitch. Win! There was that one PTA meeting that was a bit contentious, but your partner put things into perspective, and he's right: Not participating in the fundraising bake sale is not the end of the world. Now it's finally Friday night: Your partner is away on a work trip and the kids are all in bed—hopefully reading and not on their devices—and you're excited to have an evening to yourself to unwind. You grab a bag of chips from the cupboard, turn on *Ted Lasso*, and sit down to watch what happens next with Keeley and Roy. The episode finishes, and as you are getting up to go to bed, you notice the bag of chips is empty. Strange ... the family-size bag of salt-and-vinegar chips was full when you sat down. You look around to see where Roger, your cocker spaniel, is, but he's upstairs

snuggling with one of the kids. So, the dog didn't eat the chips ...
Did you really finish the whole bag? You look at your fingers, covered with oily film ... Guess it *was* you.

How does this happen? And why? The truth of it is, unconscious eating happens to all of us, maybe not necessarily with chips but some food or other. It could be the bowl of chocolate-covered almonds on your desk at work, or granola bars you keep in the car, the wrappers of which you find all over the floor mat. "How in the world did they get there? Did I really eat all those granola bars?"

We consume food all the time, but don't always notice that we're doing it. It's a great (and slightly sneaky) way our bodies make sure we survive.

Here, I'd like to make note of the difference between someone who has obesity and someone who's having a tough day. For that stressed-out person, one mindless eating episode here or there that is not part of their everyday is not what we're talking about. For someone who has obesity, someone who is consistently living below their Enough Point, they're constantly fighting their biology. Their brain is controlling how much fuel they want and making sure they get it—whether they are aware of it or not. Remember the math of biology: Food equals more fuel, and more fuel equals more energy. More energy equals yippee! The human species will continue!

To make healthier choices—and to help avoid eating out of stress, boredom, or simple habit—many weight-management programs focus on behavior change. They teach strategies for building new healthful habits, often in the context of a supportive community. And those habits can be valuable: making healthier food choices, moving more, getting better sleep, managing stress. All of these things matter for overall health and can have a significant and important impact on improving health. Additionally, changing behavior around hunger and fullness may work for some people, but it does not work for everyone. For some people, hunger is a cue they can learn to notice and use. For some, hunger persists and grows. While for others, hunger isn't something they can clearly identify at all—sometimes they don't even know what it feels like.

Oprah: I don't ever remember being hungry before. When I was a child, I just ate because it was time to eat. Later on, I was eating for all the wrong reasons. I would eat because I was upset, and it was going to calm me. Or I would eat because food was there. Or because everybody else was eating. Or I was eating to fill the void. Or I was eating to stop the food noise. Or I would just feel the need to eat . . . something, anything. It wasn't because I was hungry. In fact, I recently realized that I never allowed myself to get hungry. I literally did not know what true hunger felt like.

It's important to consider that people with obesity may not benefit in the same way or from the same behavior-change strategies; we need to understand this better. Given that people with obesity are likely living below their Enough Point, some patients report that they *are* eating in response to feeling hungry. The problem? They need to eat a lot to feel they are no longer hungry, and even more before they feel full (because they are far from their Enough Point). Patients like this who listen to their hunger actually gain weight, because their hunger persists. People with obesity have a biology that may disrupt their hunger signals, all with the goal of making sure that they gain weight and maintain that higher body fat set point.

Cognitive Load

Regardless of weight, it is important for all of us to eat as health-fully as possible and be aware of the foods we are eating. As much as is possible within our means, we want to create kitchens stocked with fruits and veggies, nutritious carbs, lean proteins, and healthy fats. This is a barrier for many, given food deserts, lack of stores with fresh veggies and fruits, lack of resources, lack of time. The goal is not perfection, just whatever is the most feasible for a person given their life circumstances. This may be frozen fruits and veggies, eggs, or cottage cheese, all examples of good sources of nutrition. When possible, eating healthfully adds joy and happiness and energy to our lives, and we feel better. We're more likely to dance to the radio, rock our shift at work, and crush that fundraising 5K when we have nutritious fuel coursing through our bodies. That said, keeping up a pantry and meal planning is challenging. Doing that with food noise? While double- and triple-checking that you're really hungry and not just bored or tired or cranky or stressed? While raising a family, holding down a job (or two), caring for aging parents, figuring out the Tetris game of after-school activities? While managing your weight in the setting of obesity without medication? It's a lot ... as I saw with my patient Nora.

Nora was in her mid-sixties, with bright hazel eyes that spar-kled when she spoke and all the charm of her Irish ancestors. She worked in a gardening store and loved helping people find just the right perennials. She had engaged in a popular weight-management program on and off throughout much of her adult life, losing weight successfully (so many times!) but always gain-ing it back. Still, she loved the in-person interaction the program offered, and sharing with others what had worked for her.

When she came to see me, she had recently regained fifty-six pounds. After discussing with me the pros and cons of medications and bariatric surgery, she elected to skip both, and try the program once again. "I'm making this my job," she told me.

I supported her in her plan because this was her choice for her life and it's what she wanted to do, but I was also concerned that she would be white-knuckling it and fighting her biology as she had many times before. Nevertheless, as health care providers we are guides in our patients' health journeys and my job is to listen, inform, and support my patients' choices because these are their lives to live. Nora left my office with a game plan.

She was determined to get down to her goal weight and get off her blood pressure medications, and she planned to devote as much time to the program as she did to her job. Over the course of a year, Nora lost sixty-eight pounds with the program. She was so happy! In the meantime, she had gotten a new pixie haircut and a new wardrobe and was getting excited for her daughter's wedding.

Every time Nora came in for a visit, we talked about what was working and what she was struggling with. I made sure she knew that if the weight ever started to creep back up, there were medications we could use to help her. "I want to do it on my own," she said. I continued to support her and I was glad she was feeling well.

For another year or so, Nora kept most of the weight off. Sometimes she came in and shared things were going well, and that her program wasn't so difficult. Other days she came in saying that she was having a tough time.

During the whole experience, Nora was using the executive part of her brain to control *every* bit of food she was eating and *exactly* how much physical activity she was doing. All of this was taking up a significant part of her day, and in some ways it seemed to dominate her life.

Despite all her work, it became harder and harder for her to control her weight. She was doing all the same things, but somehow (remember metabolic adaptation?) her vigilant routines weren't working as well. Her subconscious wasn't helping: If she gave herself even the tiniest bit of leeway, she would go off the rails. For example, one bite of a cookie led to eating six cookies. So, she told herself, in no uncertain terms: No cookies! Ever! For the rest of her life! (Ugh.) She grew frustrated and tired, and no wonder.

Defending herself from a world full of cookies was a lot of work.

I did not see Nora for several months. Then one day, she came in and had gained back all sixty-eight pounds and then some. She was so disappointed in herself. "I know you said it wouldn't be my fault if I gained back the weight, but it *is* my fault," she said. "I'm the one who let it happen. I saw it coming back, and I just let it happen."

There it was again: the blame and shame, even though it was her biology, hardwired into the weight-controlling circuits of her brain—not her—making all the decisions. But what caught my attention was the amount of time, energy, and focus she spent thinking about and planning her food. For Nora, as with so many other people, it's a significant drain on our mental resources. Even if we've decided it's impossible and not helpful to count every calorie in and calorie out with any accuracy, that doesn't mean that we aren't spending valuable time trying to choose which foods to eat, when to eat them, and how much of them to eat. Think about picking the more healthy kale chips in the chips aisle at the grocery. Way to go! Then you bring them home and have to decide how many kale chips to eat at once—ten, or the whole bag? Then you have to make an effort not to eat the more delicious corn chips your son picked out and stowed in the pantry. Then you have to decide how long until you give yourself your next salty, green, crunchy reward . . . Yes, it's very important for all of us to focus on eating healthfully, it's just a lot harder to do it while living below your Enough Point in the setting of obesity.

People who are trying to manage their obesity with diet and exercise alone take on a humongous cognitive load as they actively work to "control" their weight. Some can keep the weight off this way for extended periods of time, but, like Nora, maybe they are spending endless amounts of time and effort planning out every detail of their diet and day. Now think of all that they could be doing if they were not constantly thinking about food, not always wondering how many calories are in a handful of shredded part-skim mozzarella for an eggplant parmesan casserole. If somewhere in the back of their minds they were not thinking about really wanting to eat all the time, maybe they'd be learning Italian while making that eggplant parmesan recipe. Or maybe they would be planning a family reunion or writing the next great American novel.

But it's nearly impossible to reach for all these other goals when your attention is constantly pulled back to managing calories, cravings, and hunger. When every spare thought is hijacked by food. That's the cost of the cognitive load. You can't outthink or out-dream biology. As my colleague Dr. Lee Kaplan once summed it up: "Overeating does not cause obesity; obesity causes overeating." Bottom line, biology drives behavior.

5

From Rainbow Pills to Gila Monsters

A Brief History of Obesity Medications

Obesity is not a new disease. It did not develop within the last half century. Some of the earliest depictions of obesity come from figurines from the Paleolithic era of the Stone Age, including the Venus of Willendorf, a statuette that depicts a female figure with obesity—it dates back to thirty thousand years ago. Over twenty-five hundred years ago, Hippocrates, the father of medicine, recognized that obesity could lead to a shorter lifespan and was a harbinger of other diseases. During the Greco-Roman era (350 BCE), Egyptian pharaohs recognized and documented obesity. In 1760, Dr. Malcolm Flemyng first officially called obesity a "disease" in a publication.

Over the hundreds if not thousands of years that obesity has been recognized as impacting health, many remedies have been tried and failed: vinegar concoctions, intricate combinations of herbs and spices including cinnamon and ginger, tobacco leaves, as well as medicinal soap, use of laxatives, and intentional purging or sweating. Oh my.

Beginning in the late 1800s, with the recognition that in cases of myxedema (a very rare, life-threatening outcome of severe untreated hypothyroidism), thyroid hormone was found to increase metabolism, and people began to focus on various formulations of this hormone for weight loss. This so-called uncoupling of metabolism increases the body's generation of heat while burning off our fat supplies, but it comes at a cost. Thyroid hormone extracts began to be used to treat obesity, despite opposition from academic physicians due to the notable risks—heart palpitations, excessive sweating, loss of muscle, heart failure, and even death. Let's jump to the 1950s, when a different form of thyroid hormone, triiodothyronine (T3), was explored. Despite initial promise, T3 did not have the intended effect. That didn't deter people: The use of various forms of thyroid hormone continued into the early 1980s—until instances of death were reported.

Because metabolism and weight are deeply linked in people's minds, thyroid problems became a kind of catchall for unexplained weight change, and this persists in some of the public's minds today. As health care providers, we are often asked about this, but the innocent thyroid gland cannot be blamed for the obesity epidemic.

What other remedies were pursued? One came from a coincidental observation of French munitions factory workers during WWI. It was noted that the workers preparing a chemical compound called dinitrophenol (DNP) were losing weight. DNP was subsequently tested for weight loss in the 1930s but resulted in rapidly progressing cataracts, blindness, and even death. Given fatalities, not surprisingly in 1935, the American Medical Association (AMA) deemed it too hazardous and banned it from human use.

Amphetamines came into use for weight loss in the 1930s. Several are FDA-approved for ADHD, and one is approved for binge eating disorder. They are highly regulated, owing to their addictive properties. Unfortunately, they continue to be misused and abused, for example in the form of "meth" (methamphetamine).

Next up: rainbow pills. These came onto the scene in the 1940s. They were sold in a variety of different bright, colorful tablets and capsules (hence the name) and included a mixture of ingredients such as amphetamines, laxatives, diuretics, and thyroid hormone, as well as barbiturates, belladonna, and corticosteroids to mitigate their side effects. What a concoction! Following a Senate investigation in 1968, which identified approximately sixty deaths and multiple other severe adverse effects, rainbow pills were banned.

Other medications had short periods of use before the FDA removed them from the market for their untoward or dangerous adverse effects. These included fen-phen (fenfluramine/phentermine), which was voluntarily taken off the market in 1997 due to its link to valvular heart disease and pulmonary hypertension. Sibutramine, available from 1988 to 2010, was removed from the market for increased risk of cardiovascular disease, including stroke. Rimonabant was never approved in the US but was used in Europe from 2006 to 2008. It was taken off the market for its impact on mood, including depression and suicidality. Most recently, lorcaserin, approved in 2012, was voluntarily withdrawn from the market in 2020 for potential cancer risk.

The parade of various remedies—from vinegar drafts to rainbow pills—reads like a cautionary tale. But during much of this time, the science of obesity was not well understood, and therefore the biology could not be targeted. The desire to lose weight was there, but not the understanding of the disease of obesity or how to treat it.

Oprah: When I went to my first diet doctor in Baltimore in 1977, he put me on an amphetamine–a little black pill. It made me so hyper and speedy that I couldn't function. I actually had to come off it, and that only made me want to eat more. When I look back, I feel gratitude that it didn't cause me true lifelong harm. I remember when fen-phen came out. I never tried it, but I remember how everybody had to stop taking it because of the heart risks–but in 1977 at 148 pounds, thinking I was so overweight that I needed to do something quickly, I was desperate for a solution. Instead, that pill was one more thing that didn't work. I don't blame the medicine–as Dr. Ania explains, we didn't understand the biology back then, and so we didn't have the tools to treat obesity.

Recent History

Why do I provide this brief history of obesity medications? One reason is to understand where we came from and why certain historic barriers exist. It's no surprise that until fairly recently, there's been an extremely wary approach to various treatments for obesity, given their sordid history. Many of the older medications were discovered by serendipity. Providers and patients would notice that a medication caused weight loss as a side effect, and it would then be repurposed for that reason—a pattern that continued for many years and is now just recently beginning to change. So over those many years, health care providers were using medications that caused "weight loss," but that's not the same as treating obesity or targeting obesity biology. And because the medicines were not designed to treat obesity or target its underlying biology, there were often off-target (unwanted) effects.

It's also important to highlight that there's no magic pill, no magic shot, for obesity treatment, just as there is not one magic treatment for cancer or any other disease. There is also not just one medicine that will work for everybody or that's right for everybody. There are different types of obesities, just as there are different types of cancer or causes of high blood pressure. This means that different people will require different treatments. Some people lose a lot of weight with the new medications, whereas others will lose no weight at all. That's why your sister may have lost fifty pounds with one of the medicines, but your cousin lost ten pounds with the same medicine. Someone may have a very good blood-pressure-lowering response to a given blood pressure medication, while another person may have a more modest response.

Oprah: Understanding the science—that obesity is a disease—was a revelation. But it was even more fascinating to learn that there are different kinds of obesity. I remember a doctor on *The State of Weight* program said that one way to think about obesity is to compare it to cancer—in that it has different causes. And it's different for every person. She explained that when we talk about what influences whether someone develops obesity—it's their genes, of course, but it's also what she called "the social determinants of health." The foods you're exposed to in your environments, and things like opportunities for exercise, or stress or trauma you've experienced. For people who really struggle with obesity, we have to understand that it's not only about moving more and eating less. It's about accepting that not all bodies are the same, and as Dr. Ania just explained, each of us may respond differently to the medicines.

We know there is variability in terms of how much weight people may lose, even though most fall into a certain range. What the studies report is the average weight response. The main outcome of the studies includes the percent of body weight that is lost. The studies are designed in this way because in 2007, the FDA set a goal, which is still in place today, for approval of a medication for obesity: It must reach an average of at least 5% weight reduction. One reason the 5% threshold was chosen is that with 3–7% weight loss, there are already clear improvements in metabolic health, so a measurable benefit to patients' health. A 5% body weight reduction can, for example, improve blood pressure, decrease triglyceride levels, decrease insulin levels, and help prevent type 2 diabetes from developing.

Health care providers have used several older obesity medications for decades, all of which met this weight reduction threshold; these medications remain very useful today. Their average weight reduction is more modest than that of semaglutide or tirzepatide, but we have used them in combination for additive or perhaps in some cases synergistic weight reduction. Each one alone achieves a body weight reduction between approximately 5 to 10%—so someone who weighed three hundred pounds at baseline would on average lose somewhere between fifteen to thirty pounds with one of these medications (with some variability). So, we often use several of these medications together (sequentially, starting and adding one after another), each potentially providing an additive effect on weight and health. Given that different medications have different targets and side effects, combination therapy introduces the potential for additional weight reduction but also additional side effects. This is true of combination treatment for just about any other chronic disease. Diabetes and high blood pressure are good examples of where combination medical therapy may be required to control blood sugar or blood pressure levels, but at the cost of potentially introducing more side effects with each medication addition. Nevertheless, with education and experience, these medications are quite useful, especially when used in combination to result in additive weight reduction.

The older medications are briefly listed below and in Table 1:

- Orlistat (brand names Xenical and Alli) prevents the absorption (from the gut to the bloodstream) of some of the fat that we have eaten. In fact, when taken before meals, orlistat helps people absorb 30% less fat. It blocks an enzyme that breaks down the triglyceride fat into smaller absorbable pieces (fatty acids). The fat that is eaten but not absorbed is deposited into the toilet. Because of all the retained fat, orlistat makes stool very oily, and it oftentimes leads to oily diarrhea and an urgent need to use the bathroom. Orlistat was FDA approved in 1999. It is still used today, and can be purchased at certain doses without a prescription, but given these undesirable side effects, it is not used often (sometimes it helps relieve constipation, which can be a side effect of the other medications). Orlistat is FDA approved for ages twelve years and above.

- Naltrexone/bupropion (brand name Contrave) is a combination medication that works in the brain using two older medicines with different indications. Bupropion is approved as monotherapy for the treatment of depression (brand name Wellbutrin) and also for smoking cessation. Naltrexone is used to treat alcohol use disorder or as a rescue for opiate overdose. With fairly mild side effects, this combo has been an effective tool. Main side effects include nausea, constipation, and mood changes. This medicine was FDA approved for obesity treatment in 2014 for ages eighteen and above.

- Phentermine (brand names Adipex-P and Lomaira) has been the most commonly prescribed obesity medication in the US for years because of its low cost and efficacy. It has historically been referred to as an anorectic. Anorectics, developed in the late 1950s and used predominantly into the 1970s, are derived from amphetamines. Chemists worked to develop these medications so that they retained the appetite-suppressing effects of amphetamines but would not have the addictive properties. Although some anorectics have been pulled from the market due to dangerous side effects, phentermine has been found to be safe when used appropriately. Its main side effects include increases in heart rate or blood pressure, insomnia, and anxiety. It was approved in 1959, when the studies required to demonstrate weight reduction efficacy and safety were much shorter, only about twelve weeks. Thus, phentermine is FDA approved for short-term use only. This presents a quandary, given that obesity is a chronic disease that necessitates chronic treatment rather than short-term dosing, and many have been eager to see longer-term data for phentermine. Thanks to Dr. Jamy Ard, a professor at Wake Forest, there is now an ongoing NIH-funded trial investigating the longer-term impacts of treating obesity with phentermine. Phentermine is FDA approved for patients over sixteen years of age.

- Phentermine/topiramate (brand name Qsymia) is a combination prescription medication that works in the brain. The benefit of the topiramate component came about serendipitously. Topiramate was developed as a medication used to treat seizures and migraines, and astute neurologists noted that people in clinical trials who were treated with topiramate lost weight. A common side effect of topiramate is feeling drowsy, sometimes with brain fog, so it was combined with phentermine, which is more activating, to potentially help balance this out. Other side effects include tingling in the hands or feet, constipation, and dry mouth. Phentermine/topiramate was FDA approved as a combination in 2012 for obesity treatment for ages eighteen years and above and subsequently FDA approved in 2022 for obesity treatment for ages twelve years and above.

- Metformin (brand names include Glucophage, Glumetza, Fortamet) has been used for decades for the treatment of type 2 diabetes (FDA approved for this indication in 1994) and historically has been the first-line therapy for this disease, but it is not approved for obesity treatment. Its impact on weight is modest on average, but for some it can be more substantial. If a person has insulin resistance, polycystic ovarian syndrome, prediabetes, or diabetes, it is a logical part of a combination therapy to provide additional weight benefits and also to aid in glucose control. Its main side effects include diarrhea and bloating, which can be mitigated with slow up-titration of dose and use of the extended-release formulation of the medication rather than the immediate-release formulation.

- Liraglutide (brand name Saxenda) is a GLP-1-based medication and is one of the older, second-generation medicines. It was FDA approved in 2014 for obesity treatment for those ages eighteen and above, and in 2025 for ages twelve years and above. It's included in Table 2 on page 138 listing the NuSH-based medications.

Table 1

Molecule name	Brand name	FDA-approved indications	Mode of delivery	Frequency	Year FDA approved
Non-NuSH-based medications FDA approved for obesity treatment					
Naltrexone/bupropion	Contrave	Obesity	oral	Twice daily	2014
Orlistat	Alli, Xenical	Obesity	oral	1–3 times daily	1999
Phentermine	Adipex-P, Lomaira	Obesity	oral	1–3 times daily	1959
Phentermine/topiramate	Qsymia	Obesity	oral	Once daily	2012
Setmelanotide	IMCIVREE	Rare genetic obesity*	injection	Once daily	2020
Non-NuSH-based medications used for obesity treatment and FDA approved for other diseases					
Bupropion	Wellbutrin	Depression	oral	1–2 times daily	1985
Metformin	Glucophage, Glumetza	Type 2 diabetes	oral	1–2 times daily	1995
Topiramate	Topamax	Seizures, migraines	oral	1–2 times daily	1996, 2004

*Setmelanotide is FDA-approved for ages six years and above for proopiomelanocortin (POMC) deficiency, protein convertase subtilisin/kexin type 1 (PCSK1) deficiency, leptin receptor (LEPR) deficiency, and Bardet-Biedl syndrome (BBS). Liraglutide is included in the table listing the NuSH-based medications, but it is one of the older medications that we use today.

The Introduction of Surgery for Obesity Treatment

What about surgery? Treatment of obesity with weight-loss (bariatric and metabolic) surgery developed back in the 1950s, but the biggest advance occurred in 1994, when the first laparoscopic gastric bypass procedure was performed. Surgeons could perform the procedure with this less invasive approach, making a few small holes in the abdomen and using tiny cameras and instruments rather than opening the whole abdomen. Death rates from the procedure declined from 4 in 1,000 in 2002 to 0.6 in 1,000 in 2009, and have since decreased further to 0.03–0.2% (lower than that observed with gallbladder removal). Currently, the most common bariatric procedure performed in the United States is the sleeve gastrectomy (where the stomach is made to be the size of a banana), followed by gastric bypass (where the intestine is rerouted and the stomach is made to be the size of a walnut).

Bariatric surgery is highly effective, with patients often losing more than one hundred pounds after a given procedure. Even so, some patients may need to lose more weight to meet their health goals. So, bariatric surgery is now being paired with medications for further weight reduction, for added efficacy. The medications can be used before or added after surgical procedures to provide additional weight reduction or help prevent weight regain, which can start to occur between twelve and eighteen months after the surgical procedure. Ten-year outcomes demonstrate that on average people regain about 25% of the weight they had lost with the surgery. So, if someone loses a hundred pounds, and they maintain seventy-five pounds of weight loss, that is still very good—but now with the medications, we can prevent this weight regain and even induce additional weight reduction to help patients reach and maintain their weight and health goals.

Life Before the Highly Effective NuSH-Based Therapies

Just a few years ago, we didn't have semaglutide or tirzepatide (or the promise of all the medicines that are yet to come). Most of my patients who might benefit from more than 5 to 10% weight reduction required a combination of medications. And if they needed more substantial weight reduction, then bariatric surgery was recommended as part of the treatment for patients with more severe obesity.

To give you an example of how we treated obesity before the new medications, I'll share Ji-hye's story. Ji-hye had lost more than sixty pounds with bariatric surgery with sleeve gastrectomy over the initial six months, but then she stopped losing weight and had not reached her goal of losing ninety pounds and getting off her blood pressure medications. A middle school science teacher with a very detailed and goal-oriented mindset, she was frustrated that she had not lost more weight to reach her goal. She did feel much healthier and was continuing to walk daily, going to the gym at least once per week, and prioritizing eating protein first at every meal. Twelve months after the surgery, she began to gain some weight. At first it was just a little bit, but then her new clothes stopped fitting her about eighteen months out. She began to worry about this concerning trend, so she asked her doctor if a medication for obesity would help her.

Her doctor was reluctant to start anything at that time. This was about ten years ago, so obesity treatment was not yet in the spotlight, there was no semaglutide or tirzepatide, and he had not prescribed any obesity medications in the past. When her physician finished medical school more than forty years ago, there was no education about obesity or its treatment. The doctor advised Ji-hye to add in two more visits to the gym every week to help prevent further weight regain and to continue working with a dietitian. Ji-hye faithfully did her sets of squats and dead lifts. She joined a Zumba class and committed to doing a cycling class every Wednesday. She met with the dietitian. She continued to prioritize protein, and made sure she drank water from her fancy new water bottle throughout each day. Despite all this, the weight kept creeping back on.

Two years after her surgery, Ji-hye realized she had gained back nearly twenty-five pounds—more than a third of what she had lost in the first place. She was devastated and blamed herself. She thought she was failing, not realizing it was her biology that was strong and pushing back. She asked her doctor again about starting a medication for obesity. He agreed and started her on one of the oral combination pills (naltrexone/bupropion) and provided her with a referral to see me at the Yale Diabetes Center, where I was seeing patients for obesity treatment at that time. She responded well to naltrexone/bupropion, and once her weight plateaued, we added daily liraglutide injections. She continued to lose weight. When she plateaued again, we added metformin to help her lose that last bit. In the end, she lost more weight with the combination of these medications than she had with surgery, and with the combination of both surgical and medical therapies she achieved her weight and health goals, including normalizing her blood pressure and being able to stop her antihypertensive medications. Ji-hye was so happy that her perseverance had paid off, and with the obesity medications she felt like she was given a new life.

Medical Clues

The problem of an inadequate or even incorrect understanding of the biology of obesity made identification of medication targets a challenge. For much of history, the focus was on increasing energy expenditure (burning calories) or decreasing energy intake (appetite suppressants) rather than on recalibrating the brain's Enough Point to a healthy level. So, it is not surprising that, like many of the first- and second-generation medications, the current NuSH class of medications were discovered somewhat by serendipity.

To understand the role of hormones and obesity treatment, we need to look back to the 1900s, when researchers found that brain tumors in the area of the hypothalamus or the pituitary could lead to the development of obesity. This finding suggested that hunger and satiety were controlled by the brain and not the stomach. It was the seminal discovery of leptin in 1994 that brought forward a completely new era of obesity research. (Remember, leptin is a hormone made in fat tissue.) For the first time it was identified that a mutated gene (for leptin, *LEP*) was associated with a signal that regulated body weight. Researchers wondered if treatment could then be similar to that of type 1 diabetes, where the replacement of the missing hormone (insulin) could effectively treat the disease.

When people with congenital leptin deficiency (a very rare genetic form of severe obesity where fat tissue does not make any leptin due to a mutation in the *LEP* gene) were given leptin, they miraculously lost weight and their hunger levels normalized. Was it possible that leptin would be the answer for treating all people with obesity? Unfortunately, that has not been found to be the case. Outside of those who have true congenital leptin deficiency (who don't make any functional leptin), people with obesity generally have high levels of leptin in proportion to their amount of fat, and adding more leptin does not appear to result in weight reduction. In the meantime, researchers have been continuing to investigate various other potential roles of leptin in obesity treatment.

Nevertheless, leptin was the spark that ignited this field by providing critical information: Biology is at play, hormones are key, and fat tissue is not just an inert fuel storage site but rather very much involved in signaling to the Enough Point regions of the brain. Leptin taught us that hormones and genes or combinations of genes are involved in regulating weight. While this was incredibly exciting, progress seemed to remain somewhat slow going.

I vividly remember a conversation from many years ago that I had with a respected senior colleague from another field of medicine. We had just walked into the ornate Beaumont Room (think Hogwarts) above the Cushing/Whitney Medical Library at Yale. By way of conversation and interest, he asked about my clinical research and patient care focus. I had already started seeing patients with obesity and had begun using what are now considered to be the older first- and second-generation medications (but this was years before semaglutide or tirzepatide) and so I shared with him that I was treating patients with obesity medications. His response was "Well, those medicines don't work, and they all have side effects."

I knew he only meant to ensure I wasn't expending my energy and time on something that he did not perceive to be helpful for patients and my research, but it still felt like a slapdown. It was disheartening to me; I was junior to him and respected his opinions as an expert clinician with many years of experience. But given that I was already seeing results in my patients, I decided to tuck away this comment and keep going.

Reflecting back now, I understand the roots of his hesitation and skepticism. For years obesity was not looked upon or treated as a disease. Potentially promising therapeutics did not pan out, and failure after failure was reported in journals and the news. Medications that appeared to work would then be found to have serious and sometimes life-threatening side effects. It seemed as if nothing could work safely and effectively.

Decades ago, our understanding of obesity biology was even more limited than it is now. We were just scratching the surface, beginning to understand the biological mechanisms of how the body regulates energy stores and how this is disrupted in the setting of obesity. Even now we are in our infancy of understanding obesity biology and potential therapeutic targets—though we are learning quickly. It's important to consider that the path we've been taking for obesity treatment is similar to the early treatment development of other chronic diseases.

Let's look at diabetes for a moment as an example of understanding a disease, its treatment evolution, and the stumbles along the way. Diabetes was first described in 1550 BCE, during Egyptian times, and for thousands of years it was thought to be a disease of the kidneys, because when untreated it results in excessive urination. The excess sugar that is characteristic of diabetes needs to go somewhere and so it goes into our urine and gets peed out. It was the sweet-tasting urine (we'd prefer not to think about why someone tasted urine to confirm this) that pointed in the direction of the body's mishandling of or inability to use glucose. In 1889, two German scientists found in animal studies that removal of the pancreas resulted in high glucose levels and eventually death. About three decades later, in 1921, insulin was isolated from the pancreas as the key hormone required for the utilization of glucose. Insulin (replacing the hormone that was missing) became the first therapeutic for the treatment of diabetes in 1922. It took another three decades, until the mid- to late-1950s, before two oral therapeutic classes of diabetes medications became available. About forty years later, this was followed by the rapid development of multiple new classes starting in the mid-1990s. So, we can see that the innovations in treatment took time and were ignited and accelerated as scientific discoveries in understanding the biology of the disease were made. Notably, the understanding that there was more than one type of diabetes, requiring different treatments (i.e., type 1 diabetes requires insulin treatment, whereas the earlier stages of type 2 diabetes do not require insulin treatment), was not clarified until the 1970s, when the autoimmune basis for type 1 diabetes was elucidated. So, an incomplete understanding of the biology of diabetes or the different types of diabetes made it challenging to develop therapies to target their specific disease processes. A scientific understanding of disease biology was key to transforming the therapeutic landscape.

Let's focus in for a moment on phenformin, which was being developed in the late 1950s. Phenformin was a promising oral medication for the treatment of type 2 diabetes—that is, until it was found to increase the risk of lactic acidosis especially in people with kidney problems, and though rare, when it occurred it had fatality rates of nearly 50%. Phenformin is currently available in a few countries around the world but was pulled off the market in the United States in the late 1970s. Phenformin's tribulations ultimately did not keep metformin—phenformin's cousin in the same class of medications—from being developed and eventually becoming first-line therapy. Metformin is now the most commonly used medication for the treatment of type 2 diabetes, and it is also being investigated for its potential anticancer, anti-inflammatory, and antiaging attributes. Imagine if this class of medications had been abandoned because of what happened with phenformin—we wouldn't have metformin treatment today. The story of diabetes and phenformin offers a critical reminder about the importance of understanding the biology of any disease. A deeper understanding of the biology of obesity enables development of medications that target the underlying disease processes and will help determine the varied forms of obesity, which will require different types of treatment. Each new medication and potential therapeutic class needs to be carefully studied for both safety and efficacy, assessing risk versus benefit to patients, but missteps and setbacks should be viewed as that, rather than a complete halt to the development of potential new therapies.

A Brief History of NuSH-Based Medications Including GLP-1-Based Therapies

The landscape for obesity treatment was very different more than a decade ago. The field was still mired in the history of therapeutic pitfalls with a nascent understanding of obesity biology. There was the slow trickling of repurposed medications into treatments that individually yielded around 5 to 10% body weight reduction. The prevalence of obesity had been increasing steadily for several decades and was heralded as a global obesity epidemic by the WHO in 2000. Enter GLP-1 receptor agonists.

I mentioned liraglutide earlier. It's a GLP-1 receptor agonist, which is one type of medicine in the family or class of NuSH-based medications. Liraglutide initially came to be commercially available in 2010 as an FDA-approved treatment for type 2 diabetes. Patients who took the medication had improvements in blood sugars, but they also incidentally lost weight (this was surprising because prior to the introduction of GLP-1-based medications, weight gain was a common side effect of achieving blood sugar control with other diabetes medications). Liraglutide was not the first GLP-1-based medicine to be developed, but it was the first medication in this family to be approved by the FDA specifically for obesity treatment (in 2014), the year after obesity was declared a disease by the AMA. In retrospect, this first-of-its-kind obesity treatment from the NuSH class of medication turned out to be a consequential milestone. Namely, it ignited the development of highly effective NuSH-based medications like semaglutide and tirzepatide. But years ago, when the medication was first approved, this turning point was not yet recognized.

Liraglutide is given as a daily injection with resulting weight reduction similar to that observed with the older oral obesity medications. The burden of a daily injection, meaningful though modest weight loss, and higher cost were an issue. With the exception of specialists who were accustomed to using the older obesity medications, at that time the daily injectable therapy did not captivate the medical field's attention for the treatment of obesity. I remember my mentor Dr. Bob Sherwin and I sitting in his office, excitedly scribbling on his whiteboard, planning out research grant proposals with liraglutide as the study intervention, but clinically it was difficult to get the cost covered for obesity treatment in patients who did not already have diabetes. Now years later, liraglutide is available as a generic medication, and, as we saw with Ji-hye, it can result in meaningful weight reduction and can also be used in combination with other older medications.

Back to the development of NuSH-based therapies, and more specifically, GLP-1 receptor agonists, which were initially developed for the treatment of type 2 diabetes. By the early 2000s, there were several classes of medications already available for the treatment of type 2 diabetes, including insulin, sulfonylureas, DPP-4 inhibitors, and metformin, but there was still a need to find medications that worked to better lower blood sugars without causing them to go too low (a known side effect of both insulin and sulfonylureas).

Enter the hormones: GLP-1 and GIP. How were these discovered? These hormones were hypothesized to exist by astute clinical investigators, who more than five decades ago, noticed something interesting that happens when glucose gets into the body by intravenous (IV) infusion, directly into the bloodstream, rather than ingestion by mouth. But first you may have to know a little more about insulin. Insulin is a hormone released from the beta cells (a glucose-sensing cell type found in little balls of cells scattered across the pancreas). Insulin is secreted in response to changes in blood sugar levels, and then it instructs our body to store sugar (as glycogen!) in our organs, especially muscle. Half a century ago, scientists noted that when glucose was given by mouth, the amount of insulin released was far, far greater than if glucose was infused into a vein—even if the glucose levels in the blood were perfectly matched. So, our bodies release a lot more insulin when we eat sugar than when we have the same amount of sugar infused into our vein. Weird! Why in the world would that be? The scientists call this phenomenon the "incretin effect" and, following their curiosity, decided to study it further.

Before the discovery of the incretin effect, the beta cells were thought to be the only glucose sensors in the body. But the implications of this seeming weirdness meant that there had to be another type of cell in the gastrointestinal tract that was sensing glucose levels from food ingestion and then communicating with the glucose-sensing, insulin-secreting beta cells in the pancreas. So, how does the intestine talk to the beta cells in the pancreas to increase the amount of insulin released? A hypothesis was that a hormone secreted from glucose-sensing cells in the gut could travel through the bloodstream to reach the beta cells. So, scientists did a bunch of extractions, purifications, experiments, and analyses of intestines to eventually identify not one but two separate hormones, GLP-1 and GIP, from two separate cell types (L cells and K cells) in different parts of the intestine.

The first hormone identified, in 1973, was GIP, followed a few years later by GLP-1. Together these two hormones were termed "incretins" and could explain the incretin effect (i.e., our body releasing more insulin in response to oral rather than intravenous glucose). As it turns out, eating stimulates the release of many other hormones. Collectively, these are the nutrient-stimulated hormones (NuSHs), and include hormones like amylin and glucagon (which are not incretin hormones) as well as GLP-1 and GIP (which are the two known incretin hormones). The signaling pathways of all these NuSHs are being explored for their therapeutic roles in obesity.

So, if GIP was discovered first, then why wasn't the search for diabetes treatments focused on that hormone? (Remember, this was before they started to even consider these to be important for obesity.) Well, when scientists administered GIP hormone by itself, it had less impact on blood sugar levels than when they administered GLP-1 in the setting of diabetes. Therefore, it made sense to prioritize development of GLP-1-based molecules to treat diabetes. Years later, it was discovered that GIP stops working well when blood sugar levels have been high for too long, and high blood sugars (hyperglycemia) is exactly what happens in the setting of diabetes. However, scientists noticed that when GIP and GLP-1 were administered *together*, the resulting amount of insulin secretion was greater than with GLP-1 alone.

The rigorous, creative, and intensive work performed by teams of scientists over decades really paid off (yay, scientists!). They identified these two new hormones, which led to a therapeutic breakthrough, initially for the treatment of diabetes, then obesity, and now potentially many other related conditions.

A Very Exciting Time

I was an endocrinology fellow in training at Yale around the time the first GLP-1 receptor agonist medication, exenatide, became available for use in humans, in 2005. This medicine treated diabetes by helping to reduce blood sugar levels by stimulating more insulin secretion, but without causing low blood sugars. I was taught as a fellow that a beneficial side effect of this new medication was weight loss, as most patients with type 2 diabetes have obesity. I remember speaking with Dr. Sherwin and being very excited. Patients started to tell us they were losing some weight "without even trying." Wow!

As I mentioned earlier, at that time the medical field was slow or even resistant to treating obesity as a disease, and few thought it could be treated safely with medications. But I didn't let any of that deter me. I was always more interested in treating obesity than diabetes. Part of this was because I was just more interested in obesity as a disease, and part of it was realizing that type 2 diabetes was almost always a result of obesity. So, seeing these new medications in use and the impact on our patients' health was a watershed moment for me. Why would we not use these medications to treat obesity—a root cause of diabetes?

This was especially salient since up until that time, what I had seen during residency training were people with diabetes *gaining* weight in part due to the medications we used to lower their glucose (insulin and sulfonylureas both cause weight gain as a side effect). Why would we give people something that in the long run would make their disease worse? As endocrinologists whose field is the treatment of hormonal diseases, we naturally began to prescribe these hormone-based medications, at the time sometimes referred to as "GLP-1 mimetics" because of the way they mimic the effect of hormones. It just made sense. In those early days, the main barriers were the high cost and ensuring that our patients were comfortable with injections. We needed to educate them that GLP-1-based medications were not insulin just because they were injectable.

But there was another therapeutic hurdle for the scientists

to overcome with GLP-1 and these new GLP-1 mimetics. Namely, the hormone disappears from our bloodstream very quickly. If it disappears quickly, it cannot do its work to decrease blood sugars or help us recalibrate our body fat set point and feel like we have enough. Enter the Gila monster. Yes, the Gila monster. This is a scaly, dragon-like lizard that is found in the deserts of the Southwest US (Arizona and New Mexico). Named after the Gila River basin, the Gila monster enjoys basking in the sun and eating little rodents, birds, and snakes. Gila monsters do not get to eat very often, and so when they do, they have to be able to digest and store as many calories as possible from each meal. In fact, they eat only five to ten meals per year and store the energy as fat in their tails (for all the times in between). Their venom contains a hormone called exendin-4, which helps the reptile store every bit of energy and also enhances insulin secretion. By good fortune, it turns out that exendin-4 works very similarly to human GLP-1, but it lasts much longer. This was an important clue that these GLP-1 mimetic medications could be engineered to last longer, by making their structure similar to that of exendin-4. Believe it or not, earlier GLP-1-based medications (see Table 2 on page 138) were actually based on the molecular structure of the venom from the Gila monster.

The reason why human GLP-1 and GIP last such a short time is that there is an enzyme in our blood, called dipeptidyl peptidase-4 (DPP-4), that chews these hormones up. Scientists figured out that they could also treat diabetes by inhibiting DPP-4 and extending the life of the body's GLP-1 and GIP released into the blood following a meal. In fact, the first DPP-4 inhibitor was FDA approved for type 2 diabetes treatment in

2006, around the same time as the first GLP-1 receptor agonist, exenatide, was approved.

So, while the initial GLP-1 mimetic medication, namely exenatide, was based on the venom of the Gila monster, later medications like liraglutide resembled the structure of the GLP-1 hormone made in our human gut (but with enhancements learned from the savvy Gila monster).

Semaglutide followed next with a very similar structure to liraglutide but with additional modifications to make it last for a week. Somewhat surprisingly, making semaglutide last longer also made it a much more efficacious medication for weight reduction, opening the door to the wave of highly effective NuSH-based therapies. Next came tirzepatide, which was also designed to last for a week but was made on the structural backbone of GIP. It could bind to the GIP receptor and GLP-1 receptor, making it the first dual NuSH receptor agonist. Innovations continue to this day at a rapid pace; check out chapter 10 for a peek at what's to come. Let's talk about some of the trials that led to the FDA's approval of semaglutide and tirzepatide for the treatment of obesity.

Milestone Research Trials

The STEP 1 trial was a pivotal phase 3 study designed to specifically test semaglutide for the treatment of obesity. The results were published in February 2021 in the prestigious *The New England Journal of Medicine* (*NEJM*) with lead author Dr. John Wilding. In the trial, participants who were treated with semaglutide demonstrated an average weight reduction of about 15% over the course of sixty-eight weeks (just over a year); this degree of weight reduction had previously not been seen with any single agent. We were all very excited! But in those days, we were still in the midst of the COVID pandemic. Instead of going to giant conference halls filled with physicians, scientists, reporters, and patients to share the results, we were relegated to Zoom. Nevertheless, these key results led to the FDA's approval of semaglutide for the treatment of obesity on June 4, 2021. Semaglutide had actually been FDA approved for diabetes treatment four years earlier, in 2017, and we had already begun to use it to treat obesity when we could get it covered by insurance.

Interestingly, the endocrinologists who were using semaglutide in patients with diabetes weren't seeing the large amount of weight reduction that those of us using it in patients with obesity alone were observing. This is in fact what various trials (with semaglutide, tirzepatide, and other medicines) have now demonstrated: Specifically, participants who have obesity but who do not have diabetes (yet) lose more weight with these medications than those who already have diabetes in the setting of their obesity. The difference between the weight reduction for people with and without diabetes is about 5–7%, or about one-third less weight reduction with these medications if a patient already had diabetes. For a patient starting at 230 pounds, not having diabetes would on average result in weight loss of an additional 15 pounds versus for someone who already had diabetes. This is the difference between weighing 210 versus 195 pounds. Not a negligible difference. So for those of us who were treating patients with obesity rather than patients who already had diabetes, we realized early on that this would be a highly effective medication, and we were very excited!

Let's back up to June 2020, when the STEP 1 trial top-line results were first revealed. (At the end of a study, before a trial goes through the process of being written up and reviewed by experts in the field for eventual publication, a predetermined set of results gets released to the world: the top-line results.) I remember hearing these early results, showing remarkable weight reduction, during the early days of the COVID pandemic, while sitting on Zoom. It felt like being in a padded room and wanting to shout to the world that everything about treating obesity and the health of millions of people and the future of medicine were about to change, but no one could hear. Although the results were extremely impressive—for the first time reaching the 15% body weight reduction threshold with a single agent (an average of thirty-two pounds in participants of the STEP 1 trial)—it took time for the world to recognize what had just occurred. And it was just the beginning.

While those results were being disclosed, at Yale and other sites around the world, we were seeing participants who had enrolled in the pivotal SURMOUNT-1 phase 3 trial of tirzepatide for obesity treatment. The purpose of this trial was to determine if there was an additional benefit for treating obesity by activating *both* the GLP-1 *and* GIP receptors. We had started the trial in December 2019; not ideal timing given the unknown looming COVID-19 pandemic. Somehow we and the other sites were able to continue supporting participants throughout the pandemic (no small feat)—keeping the participants in the study safe and on their weekly doses of tirzepatide or placebo.

Leading the Yale site of the study, I was blinded to the outcome, meaning I was not allowed to see the results in my center or any other. I knew some of our participants had lost more weight than I had seen previously with just one medicine. I had a feeling that these results would be impressive. Alice was one of those participants.

I will never forget the cloudy, cool morning of April 28, 2022. I was looking for my white coat because later that day, I was going to be seeing patients together with another clinician at the Yale Diabetes Center. At that time, the obesity clinic was still combined with the diabetes clinic on the third floor of the Dana Clinic Building. My phone started buzzing when the top-line results came out—nearly 23% body weight loss in seventy-two weeks. Astonishing!

Then things got crazy. With myself as lead author, the SURMOUNT-1 team of coauthors, scientists, and biostatisticians, and I would have to review, analyze, and interpret the data and prepare the figures. I'd need to write the scientific manuscript, edit and revise with my coauthors' input, coordinate the submission to the *NEJM*, and organize a simultaneous presentation at the American Diabetes Association's (ADA) Scientific Sessions. Hours and hours on Zoom and phone calls, not to mention hours of writing. The manuscript would have to be reviewed by several anonymous experts in the field, edited and reviewed again, edited again, reviewed again, and edited again—with the goal of simultaneous publication with the ADA's Scientific Sessions on June 4, 2022. All this in just six weeks!

It was a notable meeting of the ADA for another reason: This was the first time the association was open to focusing on obesity treatment as well as diabetes research. Previously, the ADA and other associations and societies had not been interested in focusing on obesity, which, in 1981, led to a group of doctors splintering off and establishing the North American Association for the Study of Obesity (now called The Obesity Society, or TOS). But now endocrinologists and diabetes specialists were beginning to recognize and acknowledge that obesity research was critical to diabetes. It was as if the winds were beginning to shift and all of a sudden everyone had simultaneously begun to realize that treating obesity was key to helping millions of people around the world.

I was thrilled.

As I wrote the manuscript, what kept me centered was thinking about all the patients who could be affected and how their health and lives could and would be transformed. I am honored to have had the opportunity to work closely with Dr. Julie Ingelfinger, the deputy editor at *NEJM*, and with Dr. Marlon Pragnell from the ADA, in the exciting, yet frenetic, process. This was going to be the first major scientific meeting in our field since the pandemic, and because the meeting was still hybrid, we did not know if people would show up in person. A big room that could fit several thousand people was booked just in case. I thought a lot about Alice and how her life had changed by losing ninety pounds over the course of the trial. This was much more than just a manuscript about a highly effective medication. This was an opportunity for the medical community to understand and embrace that we now had effective tools to treat obesity. That the tools were targeting the biology of obesity. That treating obesity effectively would change our patients' lives and health as well as the face of medicine.

June 4 came before we knew it. I had averaged three hours of sleep a night for those six weeks. None of us on the team had slept much during that time. We'd also had to put together the slide presentation equally as fast. Dr. Louis (Lou) Aronne from Weill Cornell Medicine was set to present the study background, which provided the context for understanding the results, but the day before, we learned that he had contracted COVID. He was feeling okay but, of course, couldn't be there in person. The rest of us made it to balmy, humid New Orleans for the ADA's eighty-second Scientific Sessions meeting. The night before we were set to present, our team practiced into the wee hours. Dedicated Dr. Aronne, literally feverish, joined in virtually from his home to practice with us by Zoom. Things were coming together as we left our practice session to catch a power nap before the presentation in the morning.

It wasn't until I woke up that morning that I knew how I would open the presentation, how I would capture the audience of mostly diabetologists. I knew this was too important for our patients not to get it just right. I quickly remade my opening slides as my incredibly supportive husband brought me a cappuccino. His day job is as a physician-scientist endocrinologist at Yale, but his self-defined job for those six weeks was to always make sure I had coffee and supportive hugs. All of us were masked walking into the convention center. It was already humid outside, and we were jolted awake by the bracing air-conditioning. We patiently waited in the sparse line to have our temperature checked before we were allowed passage. Our palms were slimy from the pumps of hand sanitizer. Would we be speaking to an empty room?

We were ready. We had a dream team. Our chairs were Dr. Donna Ryan, from Pennington Biomedical Research Center—the mother of obesity medicine, and a mentee of internationally recognized researcher and grandfather of obesity medicine Dr. George Bray—and Dr. Jamy Ard, from Wake Forest University School of Medicine, whose calmness and sense of humor in the face of stressful situations is second to none. Steadfast Dr. Aronne would be presenting from his home; he still managed to put on a suit jacket and tie despite a fever of 102°F. The rest of us were in person. Dr. Sean Wharton, from the Wharton Medical Clinic, would set us up beautifully by describing the study design and participants. Dr. Sriram Machineni, from the University of North Carolina, would be presenting the safety results with his steady timbre. And Dr. Lee Kaplan, from Harvard Medical School, would share his deeply thoughtful big-picture view, framing the results within the context of current available treatments and bringing it all home. I was to present the weight-loss efficacy results in between Drs. Wharton and Machineni. Already in the audience were the science drug discovery team and a coauthor with whom I had spent long nights perfecting every word of the manuscript. People started crowding in. It was going to be standing room only.

Drs. Aronne and Wharton presented their parts; now it was my turn to present the efficacy results. I walked up the steps to the podium. It was a large ballroom, and the entire audience was waiting on edge to hear what I was about to share. I smiled, took a deep breath, and exhaled. I began, "Why are we all here today?" I paused for a long time, letting the impact of the question reverberate in all our minds. You could hear a pin drop; this was not the typical way to begin a presentation of the main results at a scientific symposium.

I continued, "Whether you're a clinician, a scientist, a patient, we're all here with one common goal. We're all here because we want to help patients lead healthier lives. And now we have the opportunity to do so, by treating obesity. By treating the disease that underlies over two hundred other diseases, including diabetes." Over the next twenty minutes, I presented the results from the SURMOUNT-1 trial. The data spoke for itself: Patients lost on average more than 22% of their body weight; the participant group averaged fifty-two pounds of weight loss with seventy-two weeks of treatment with tirzepatide. Their blood pressure improved. Their cholesterol improved. Their blood sugars improved. Their health improved. Some felt, as did Alice, that their whole lives had improved.

It was as if the winds shifted that day in the room filled with endocrinologists, diabetologists, scientists, patients, and reporters. The data was so compelling, so clear. I ended with Alice's words: "It's just as easy to lose weight as it ever was to gain weight."

Alice captured the biology of obesity in that one sentence, the biology as she experienced it. The lead-up to that moment was a blur, especially after having slept only a few hours a night during the preceding weeks. But when I showed those first slides from the podium and heard the gasps of amazement in the otherwise complete stillness of the packed room, it was worth it. From my perspective, that moment in time was absolutely pivotal for our patients with obesity. The data spoke for itself: We could now effectively and safely treat obesity and, in so doing, improve our patients' lives and health while also potentially preventing, mitigating, and treating hundreds of other diseases.

I finished speaking, and as I walked offstage, our session co-chair Dr. Ard said, "Wow, if you're not excited, check your pulse!"

6

Enough Is Enough (Finally)

Starting the Medications

There are transformative moments in medicine—discoveries that not only save lives but reshape how we understand disease. Penicillin, the first antibiotic, has saved an estimated 500 million lives since its accidental discovery in a mold-ridden petri dish in 1928. It taught us how to target infectious bacteria. Insulin was another breakthrough: the first peptide hormone purified for human use and the first protein ever sequenced. It transformed the lives of people with type 1 diabetes, turning a once-fatal diagnosis into a manageable condition. Now, we're at another watershed moment. The emergence of highly effective obesity medications is transforming patient lives through treatment and disease understanding. These therapies are revealing the underlying biology of obesity and helping us target it more precisely. That's what happened with the introduction of semaglutide and tirzepatide.

The media frenzy that followed the tirzepatide SURMOUNT-1

symposium at the ADA's Scientific Sessions and the manuscript publication in *NEJM* was astounding and continued for weeks. I was certainly exhausted and overwhelmed, as were my colleagues.

We were also excited. Finally, our patients were going to be able to get the effective and safe treatments they needed for obesity, with NuSH-based medications opening that door wide open. But as with all new opportunities, there were also challenges ahead. Over the ensuing months, health care providers started becoming more accustomed to prescribing the medications, and patients became more accustomed to asking for them. Semaglutide and tirzepatide were prescribed to people with obesity in addition to those with diabetes. In the trials for people with obesity, semaglutide on average had reached a weight-loss efficacy of just over 15%, and tirzepatide over 22%. For people with diabetes and obesity, semaglutide reached on average nearly 10% body weight reduction, and tirzepatide reached nearly 15%. Those results were all very encouraging and created a lot of interest and use.

But shortages ensued in 2022. The need for these medications was so great that the companies could not manufacture enough. Initially some insurance companies covered the cost, then they didn't, and the out-of-pocket costs were out of reach for many if not most people. It was heartbreaking to experience this with my patients who had been waiting for better treatments for years.

Of course, not everyone was interested in taking one of these medications or treating their obesity, but still, more than half of Americans qualified for one of these two medications. Additionally, in contrast to most diabetes medications, which can be slowly adjusted up to the exact needed dose by using a multi-dose injector pen, the obesity medications were being placed in single-dose injector devices. Overall, single-dose injector devices, though simple for patients to use, are expensive and resource-consuming—and add more plastic waste to our struggling planet. Single-dose injectors also create a situation where it is quite difficult to adjust the dose if side effects occur. If a patient needs a lower dose, doctors can't advise them to dial back the dose (as on a multi-dose injector pen) and take less of the medicine. Instead, those providers have to prescribe a new four-pack of single-dose injectors, which quite often needs approval from the patient's insurance company and is sometimes denied given that the patient was just dispensed a four-pack of the higher dose from their pharmacy. But if a patient can't tolerate the higher dose they were just dispensed, what are they to do? A situation that would easily be solved if the medicine came in a multi-dose injector pen versus a single-dose injector device. During these shortages, people were sometimes prescribed doses that were higher than the lowest starting doses, leading to otherwise preventable side effects. Early on in the shortage, the issue wasn't that there was not enough semaglutide; it was that there was insufficient semaglutide in the single-dose injector devices. The medication shortages lasted until 2024 for tirzepatide and 2025 for semaglutide. Seeing patients regain fifty, sixty, eighty pounds after losing access to a medication, whether due to a shortage or loss of insurance coverage, was and continues to be egregious and heartbreaking.

Hormones Are Key

From these early months until today, there have been a lot of questions as to how these medications work. To answer these questions, we need to go back to the internal feedback loops of energy and fat store regulation in the brain and the role hormones play in that constant dialogue between the body and the brain.

As noted, GLP-1s are hormones made by our bodies; they are not the medications themselves. The medications, on the other hand, *look* similar to the hormones. They *behave* similarly to hormones, but they are not the hormones themselves. The medicines are made in a lab by chemists to imitate hormones and are administered at doses that are much higher than what our bodies would ever make and are also made to last a lot longer.

Another way to think of hormones is as keys. Each type of key (a hormone) fits a specific lock (a receptor) that then enables opening a door to deliver a message. If a certain organ has that specific lock (receptor), the key opens the lock and works in that organ. Without that lock (receptor), the hormone (key) will not work in that particular organ or tissue. Our bodies are pretty cool. The new medicines target the same locks as our hormones, but they target *more* locks in our bodies and brains, and they target them for *longer.*

Here's why: Some of our hormones last for only a short time in our bodies. In fact, the half-life of our bodies' GLP-1 hormone is one to two minutes. The half-life of GIP is five to seven minutes. This means that when we eat, we secrete GLP-1, GIP, and other NuSHs, and these hormones signal to our brain that we're full. But in the time it takes you to finish the food on your plate (depending on how fast you eat), the levels of those hormones made by your body are going down. You do secrete more GLP-1 and GIP as you keep on eating, but relatively soon after you finish your meal, the receptors in your brain are no longer getting the signal that you're still eating and filling up with nutrients. So, you may start getting hungry again, perhaps even before you've stepped away from the table. Or you may finish dinner and feel like you're not really full at all.

Some supersmart chemists thought to themselves, "What if there was a way we could target these receptors for longer?" In other words, what if we could keep the locks—the ones that tell our bodies we're filling up or full—open for longer?

To do that, they initially focused on the pancreas. As mentioned, when these chemists began their work, they were primarily interested in treating diabetes, not obesity. They knew that GLP-1, GIP, and other hormones broke down quickly. And they knew that the reason they broke down so fast was because of the enzyme dipeptidyl peptidase-4, or DPP-4.

Eureka! Remember the Gila monster? Its saliva has the hormone exendin-4, which is similar to human GLP-1 but resistant to the DPP-4 enzyme that breaks down the GLP-1 hormone. So the smart scientists learned from the Gila monster and created peptides that were more resistant to DPP-4. How does this work? Picture a necklace strung with glass beads: The scientists replaced some of the glass beads with metal beads that wouldn't break or chip, no matter if you dropped the necklace, stepped on it with your heel, or, in the case of our biology, faced a bunch of DPP-4s. Thus, these new peptides were more durable. The result was, drum roll . . . that the effect on the body and brain lasted much, much longer and therefore had a greater overall effect on the patient's biology, including the biology that is controlled by the brain.

These peptides became the new NuSH-based medications. And just as the chemists predicted, they have half-lives of not just minutes but days—in some cases many days. Semaglutide's half-life is about 168 hours (seven days) and tirzepatide's half-life is about 120 hours (five days). There are new medications in development that last even longer—one in phase 3 of development is MariTide, which has a half-life of twenty-one days. No matter how you count it, these medicines create a huge advantage over the few minutes of the naturally occurring NuSHs in terms of appetite and of regulating our Enough Point. Specifically, because these peptides last so much longer than the body's hormones, they also get into more helpful places, like our brains.

Our natural hormones get into the brain, and some are even produced in the brain. With regard to the medicines, we're still not sure exactly how they communicate to our brains to turn down the Enough Point. But they do seem to communicate, "Hey! Reduce the fuel you're storing. You'll be just fine. You won't starve. You'll survive! You're okay!" And with that message, maybe the pasta fork stops twirling. We don't feel like we need to take another bite of food.

This is wonderful news! Our brains now see that we need less fuel, so our bodies stop taking in so much of it. But in order for our brains to keep our thermostats at this lower body fat set point, they need the medicines, or a form of treatment that recalibrates the Enough Point, *all the time*. At least from what we're seeing now, without the medicine, the brain flips back to its old body fat set point: "Gimme more fuel, gimme more banana cream pudding, gimme more chicken fajitas with a large side of sour cream and guac." There is variability in how quickly people gain back the weight and how much weight they gain back, but on average the weight is regained.

Remember that the same is true for any chronic disease (i.e., one without a cure). High blood pressure is a chronic disease. Medications control it, but only if you take them! The medicines don't work if they're still in the bottle or the syringe. They must be in your body all the time in order to work all the time. Obesity is no different. The other thing to remember is that under no circumstances would our bodies ever make this much of a given hormone (GLP-1, GIP, or any other) or one that would last as long as the medications. With these medications, we are not giving back to our bodies what they are deficient in; instead, we are giving our bodies medications that activate the biological pathways of these naturally occurring hormones to a greater extent and for longer.

The Nitty-Gritty (as of Now)

If you've read this far, hopefully you have a clearer understanding of how the medicines work in general. Now let's move on to the nitty-gritty of specific medicines. We see them in the newsstand advertisements, on social media, and hear about them from our doctors, neighbors, family members, and friends: She's on this, he's on that, they're taking this and that. Everybody has an opinion—which can be confusing.

Here's a table of the current FDA-approved NuSH-based medications available in the US in 2025:

Table 2

Molecule name	Brand name	Target	FDA-approved indications	Mode of delivery	Frequency	Initial Year FDA approved
NuSH-based medications (third generation)						
Semaglutide	Wegovy	GLP-1 receptor	Obesity, MASH‡, CVD*	Injection	Weekly	2021
Semaglutide	Ozempic	GLP-1 receptor	Type 2 diabetes	Injection	Weekly	2017

Semaglutide	Rybelsus	GLP-1 receptor	Type 2 diabetes	Oral	Daily	2019
Tirzepatide	Zepbound	GIP and GLP-1 receptors	Obesity, OSA†	Injection	Weekly	2023
Tirzepatide	Mounjaro	GIP and GLP-1 receptors	Type 2 diabetes	Injection	Weekly	2022
NuSH-based medications (second generation)						
Dulaglutide	Trulicity	GLP-1 receptor	Type 2 diabetes	Injection	Weekly	2014
Liraglutide**	Saxenda	GLP-1 receptor	Obesity	Injection	Daily	2014
Liraglutide**	Victoza	GLP-1 receptor	Type 2 diabetes	Injection	Daily	2010
NuSH-based medications (first generation)						
Exenatide**	Byetta	GLP-1 receptor	Type 2 diabetes	Injection	Twice daily	2005
Exenatide**	Bydureon	GLP-1 receptor	Type 2 diabetes	Injection	Weekly	2012

NuSH—nutrient-stimulated hormone
*CVD—cardiovascular disease—semaglutide is also approved to reduce the risk
of major adverse CV events (CV death, nonfatal myocardial infarction, or nonfatal
stroke) in adults with established CV disease and obesity; note: dulaglutide, liraglutide,
and semaglutide also have an FDA indication of CV disease risk reduction in persons with
diabetes
†OSA—obstructive sleep apnea—tirzepatide is also approved for moderate to severe OSA
‡MASH—metabolic-associated steatohepatitis
**Generic liraglutide and short-acting exenatide are available; Byetta and Bydureon were
discontinued in 2024

Looking at this table, you may have noticed a few things: Different brand-name medications are actually the same molecule (the same peptide medicine). Surprise, surprise: Molecules with the same name all work the same way! At the end of the day, Zepbound and Mounjaro are the same molecule (peptide)—tirzepatide. Wegovy, Ozempic, and Rybelsus are the same molecule (peptide)—semaglutide. Why your provider prescribes one over the other usually has to do with your insurance coverage for these medications for obesity and obesity-related diseases, and the most cost-effective way of providing you with treatment.

You probably also saw that under "mode of delivery," most are injectables. Currently, many of these treatments require an injection because our digestive enzymes love to gobble everything up, especially peptides—that's their job! So, when we take peptides orally, our stomach juices chew up those peptide molecules before they are able to perform their function. To counteract this, you need to take *more* of the peptides to do the same job. So, the dose of a peptide administered orally is higher than the dose that is used when administered by injection if the same efficacy is sought. That is why the dose of oral semaglutide is higher than the dose of injectable semaglutide.

You'll also see that right now, all the molecules on the list are peptides—semaglutide, tirzepatide, liraglutide, dulaglutide, and exenatide (that little "-tide" suffix is a handy hint that connotes a peptide in the NuSH-based class of medicines). Down the road there will also be NuSHs that are small molecules (not peptides) that can be administered orally and are not chewed up by our digestive juices (hooray!). These are in development and will have a different ending: "-glipron," as in orforglipron, rather than "-tide."

You may have also noticed in the table that the GLP-1 receptor is included as a target for all the current approved medications, but tirzepatide also targets the GIP receptor. Down the road, there will be many other new medications that target different NuSH receptors, like amylin, PYY, and glucagon receptors. These new NuSH-based medications will be very useful, because targeting different receptors allows us to treat different biological mechanisms, thus hopefully different types of obesities and obesity-related conditions.

There are different types of obesity—we just don't know how to differentiate them as yet—and these will likely require different forms of treatment. Not everyone responds to the current medications, some people don't lose any weight, and, although rare, some people do have persistent side effects to GLP-1-based medications, so we need more choices and options for everyone. As we've already discussed, there are many, many different types of obesities, so your obesity may not be the same as your neighbor's obesity or even your mother's obesity. We need different medicines and therapies to treat all the different types of obesities.

Another thing you may have noticed about the table is that most of these medications are approved for type 2 diabetes, but not always for obesity. As we discussed, this class of medications was initially developed for type 2 diabetes and then some went on to be developed for obesity treatment. Most of these medications are currently FDA approved for adults who are at least eighteen years old. Additionally, semaglutide and liraglutide are both approved for those ages twelve and above for obesity. Liraglutide and dulaglutide are both FDA approved for ages ten and above for type 2 diabetes. Trials with tirzepatide are ongoing in youth.

Old and New Medicines in Practice

When Swati initially came to see me nine years ago, before the newer NuSH medications, she was eighteen years old and interested in getting a degree in health care administration. She had a positive "let's do this" energy about her, and she brightened the mood anytime she walked into a room. She and her family all lived in larger bodies, so she was seemingly shielded, or had shielded herself, from negative emotions of shame or self-blame. However, she could not lose and keep the weight off; despite her best efforts, her BMI was over 50 kg/m² (severe obesity). She already had pre-diabetes and sleep apnea. Her mother and father and most of her grandparents had type 2 diabetes. She wanted to follow in their footsteps, but not in terms of diabetes.

Swati was teary when we first spoke about the facts regarding biology, but then she was all in to create and follow a treatment plan. "Okay, sounds great," she said. She wanted to try medications before pursuing surgery, to see how far she could get, then circle back around to see if surgery was her next best option. She started taking metformin, walking more, focusing on choosing the middle healthy choice, rather than an all-or-nothing way of eating (it turns out, a life of undressed salads is pretty boring!). She lost fifteen pounds and then plateaued, so we added liraglutide. She diligently took the injection every day, and we slowly increased the dose. Aside from slight nausea and occasional diarrhea after eating samosas, she did not have significant side effects, which was wonderful. She continued on this path, and over the course of about eighteen months she lost more weight. Her BMI was now in the mid-to-low-40s—a great response.

At that point, her weight plateaued once more. We added the generic medications naltrexone and bupropion, and this really helped. Her BMI decreased into the 30s. With every successful visit, she flashed me another understated, shy smile—but I could tell she was incredibly happy with her results. She continued to take all four medications, and lost over 130 pounds. "I feel great!" Swati said in her soft-spoken voice. She was a woman of few words, but just kept on doing what she needed to do.

When semaglutide was FDA approved, we decided to switch her from liraglutide to semaglutide. This switch would enable her to go from a once-daily (liraglutide) to a once-weekly injection (semaglutide). Because semaglutide was more efficacious than liraglutide, we started to lower the doses of the naltrexone and bupropion as we increased the dose of semaglutide. Eventually, over the course of about three and a half years, she lost more than 150 pounds and reached a BMI of 25. Her obstructive sleep apnea resolved, and her prediabetes went into remission.

Swati's story is inspiring—and indicative of how much work it takes to get healthy, at every stage. She was young yet already exhibiting downstream obesity-related diseases including sleep apnea and elevated blood sugar levels in the setting of prediabetes. She started with a firm belief in the process, stayed consistent with her treatment, kept on going with all the hard work, and remained positive that she would maintain the weight as long as she kept going with treatment. She did finish that health care administration degree, and kept on living her life—healthier, more confident, and positive in all she did. I found myself beaming during Swati's appointments too, so glad to see her happy and healthy.

To be clear, medications are not the right choice for everyone. As mentioned earlier, when we doctors or health care providers think about using medications (or any form of treatment), we always take into account the benefits versus the harms. So, when I'm exploring treatment for a patient, I consider all the information we have: How is obesity impacting that patient now? How may it affect their health later? Does it increase their risk for other diseases?

Based on this, we determine if a medicine is worth the risk, and which medicine that may be. What do I mean by risk? Well, there is no medicine, no treatment, that has zero risk. In the case of these medications, there are common side effects and rare side effects (I discuss these in chapter 9). There is no way to make the risk of side effects zero. I discuss this in detail with my patients, always including them in the decision-making about their treatment and care.

We also discuss the risk of *not* treating. If someone has uncontrolled diabetes for decades, they can develop heart disease and nerve problems. Diabetes is the number one cause of blindness and kidney failure in the United States. It's similar to obesity in that *not* treating it can have many detrimental effects on health and quality of life. Severe obesity (BMI ≥ 40 kg/m^2) shortens life expectancy by as much as fourteen years. Why? Because in addition to being a disease in and of itself, obesity leads to obesity-related diseases and complications from obesity, including type 2 diabetes, high blood pressure, high cholesterol, and certain types of cancers, including colon cancer, thyroid cancer, and breast cancer in postmenopausal women. That's just a glimpse of the potential health problems: As noted earlier, there are over two hundred obesity-related diseases or obesity complications. But if we treat obesity earlier, these diseases can potentially be prevented or addressed by treating the underlying or root cause—the obesity itself.

Yolanda, a talkative and engaging woman in her fifties, was a mother of four, with two Chihuahuas. She loved having all her extended family over to her home every Sunday for festive family dinners that included multiple generations, home-cooked empanadas, and lots of love. She came to me interested in seeing what our clinical program could offer and what her options were, and curious to learn more about the medications. She had class 3 obesity (BMI $\geq$40 kg/m^2) and had continued to steadily gain weight over time. She also had prediabetes, along with high blood pressure that was well controlled. Her mother had had diabetes and was on dialysis due to kidney failure. Yolanda had been working with a dietitian for several years. She took cooking classes and walked daily with her dogs. She had tried everything to lose weight—even the "one grapefruit a day" diet—to no avail.

Yolanda and I discussed medications and bariatric surgery, including the pros and cons of both. She was not interested in surgery, nor did she want to take anything injectable. We discussed some of the older medications that were in pill form, but the potential side effects of all the medications concerned her. At the end of the initial visit, Yolanda decided to hold off on medications. She wanted to continue to "try on her own."

In Yolanda's case, this was challenging. She'd seen what can happen when obesity goes untreated, as happened with her mother, but for her, the possible risks of using the medications outweighed the potential benefits; she wanted to be certain that she would not have nausea or develop gallstones. Since both can happen, even if the latter is rare, there was no such guarantee. Feeling that the disease was her own fault, and having watched her mother inject insulin for years, she was reluctant to start any type of injections. Patient autonomy is incredibly important. Just as a patient can choose not to have medical treatment for other diseases, whether it's high blood pressure, high cholesterol, or diabetes, patients can decide whether or not they would like to pursue treatment for their obesity, what type of treatment, and when.

Oprah understands what my hesitant patients are going through.

Oprah: Back in 2018, as I mentioned, a friend was at the house and told me they were on this new weight-loss drug that they shot into their stomach. I was like, "Are you kidding? Not me. I'm not going to be shooting anything into my stomach." Gayle and I were sitting at the table, and we both said, "No, I'd never do that!" But I realize now, that is such antiquated thinking–to still be in the space of "You should be able to do it yourself" or "You shouldn't be taking the drug from diabetics." First of all, you can't do it yourself–at least not long-term–and second, you're not taking drugs from others. These are new medicines for us. In fact, as Dr. Ania says, many of these drugs that are being developed work better in terms of weight loss for people who do not yet have diabetes.

I was a reluctant patient. I was like those folks back in the day who said, "Well, I'm gonna hold on to my horse. I don't care what kind of automobiles they get. I'm still keeping old Dusty in the stable, doggone it." Or the folks who said, "Actually, I prefer candles, because I don't know what this electricity's going to do." I was going to hold on to my horse–even though he couldn't get me where I needed to go. I was going to hold on to the candles–even though they might burn down my house. But I've learned that this modern medicine is changing people's lives, and it's saving people's lives. I'm always so happy to hear of people who, like me, were hesitant to try the medications, then change their minds and discover what the medicines can do for them.

Changing Minds

Two clinic visits later, Yolanda did decide to start one of the medications. To successfully do this, we had to address her roadblocks: For her, one barrier was that she felt that obesity was her fault. So, what did we do? You guessed it—over the next few visits, we talked about biology! Then we addressed another barrier: her fear of needles, which was rooted in watching her mother take insulin for diabetes and eventually develop kidney failure. As we dove into a better understanding of these barriers to treatment and care, she began to understand that obesity was not something that she chose, that it was not her fault, and that needles did not equate to having to take insulin or developing the negative downstream effects of diabetes. We talked about the side effects, the more common ones and the rare ones, so that she could make an informed decision about her treatment and care. She became open to trying to see if a medicine could help her treat her obesity. We discussed the older medications again to give her an oral option. In the end she decided to try one of the new weekly injectables. Her niece had tried one, and was doing well without side effects. She also felt reassured after our discussions. Well, it turns out that Yolanda happens to be a super responder to one of the medicines. She needs just the very lowest dose once a week, and has already lost forty-seven pounds. She continues to see me in clinic every few months and hasn't experienced any significant side effects. Recently she shared with me that she is happy that she did not feel pressured to start a medication, and that she did it on her own time when she felt comfortable to do so.

Decisions, Decisions

We've talked about the options, and I've shared stories of how these medicines have changed lives. But you're probably still wondering: Are medications right for you? If you have early obesity (i.e., you have not had obesity for a long time) and you do not store a lot of extra fat (proxy measure as weight or BMI), then perhaps in your deliberations the risk of the medications outweighs the potential benefit. Or perhaps although you are early in the disease process you see what has happened with family members with obesity over the years and you are more eager to start a medication earlier to prevent some of the issues they have faced. If you have had obesity for some time, have tried various other methods for losing and maintaining weight reduction and nothing seems to work, then perhaps you are in a place where the medications are a potential next therapeutic option that you would like to try to treat your obesity. Perhaps you're already ready.

Guidelines are currently being written and refined as to when to start treatment, and for whom. For years, a BMI of ≥ 30 kg/m^2 or a BMI of ≥ 27 kg/m^2 with a weight-related disease (such as high cholesterol, high blood pressure, etc.) has been the general guidance for initiating these medications, but this is changing in real time as we accrue more evidence through research studies. Most agree that BMI is insufficient to use in isolation and should be paired with other measures of the disease, both in terms of identifying the disease and following treatment response.

Here's what I advise patients who come to see me in my clinic: Let's discuss—and understand—the pros and cons. These medicines are not short-term "weight-loss drugs." They are medications to treat the chronic disease of obesity. They are not a magic pill or shot that will cure your obesity. They are powerful tools that we as health care providers need to respect. If the risk of not treating obesity outweighs the risk of treating it, then the medications may be part of your treatment plan.

Who may be eligible for these medications is changing as I

write. Up until now, BMI has been used to characterize obesity. The World Health Organization (WHO) set BMI criteria as follows:

Underweight: BMI <18.5 kg/m²

"Normal" Weight: BMI 18.5–24.9 kg/m² (if most people have a BMI of >25, then what is "normal"?)

Overweight: BMI 25–29.9 kg/m² (some people call this "pre-obesity," mirroring "prediabetes")

Obesity*: BMI ≥30 kg/m²

Class 1 obesity: BMI 30–34.9 kg/m²

Class 2 obesity: BMI 35–39.9 kg/m²

Class 3 obesity: BMI ≥40 kg/m²—sometimes termed "severe obesity"

*For Asian individuals, obesity is defined with a lower BMI. The World Health Organization (WHO) Asian BMI classification:
Overweight: BMI 23–27.4 kg/m²
Obesity: BMI ≥27.5 kg/m²
Note: for certain populations in Asia the BMI cutoffs for obesity are even lower.

But does a BMI of ≥30 kg/m² really mean you have obesity? For most, probably yes. But remember, it's a simple equation based on weight and height—it doesn't take into account fat mass or fat distribution. If you are an athlete or bodybuilder, your BMI does not reflect fat stores in the same way, because you have more muscle mass. For example, Arnold Schwarzenegger's BMI was estimated to be just above 30 kg/m² at his peak physique—we would not assess him, in *The Terminator*, to have obesity. Most of us are not Arnold Schwarzenegger, but this underscores the point that BMI does not directly tell us about fat amount or distribution (where we store it). So even though most of us likely do not have the physique of Arnold Schwarzenegger, we need to identify additional and better ways to measure and assess obesity.

So back to who meets the criteria for these medications according to the FDA. Until recently, the medication package insert (the information the FDA communicates to the prescribers about medications) stated that the criteria for use of these medications was a BMI of ≥ 30 kg/m^2 or a BMI of ≥ 27 kg/m^2 with an obesity-related disease. If a person has type 2 diabetes, there is no BMI cutoff for the GLP-1 based medications, which help regulate blood sugar levels, regardless of weight. Recently, the FDA package inserts stopped including specific BMI cutoffs; rather, the inserts state that the indication is for people "with obesity or with overweight in the presence of at least one weight-related condition." So, the criteria is in flux, and that's a good thing: We are working to try to determine the optimal way to diagnose and categorize obesity, and that will take continued research to provide the FDA with the data it needs to make its decisions.

The FDA makes its careful decisions about whether or not to approve a medicine and whom that medicine should be approved for by assessing risk versus benefit for each new compound in development. It can do so only by reviewing all available data. What does this data include? There is data on safety (is it safe to take, or are there toxic effects?), tolerability (what are the side effects, and are they mainly mild-to-moderate and tolerable to the patient?), and efficacy (how well does it address the target outcome of a particular disease?).

Here is where clinical trials come in. This is what I do as a physician-scientist conducting clinical research: gathering data about a range of people, looking at a different medication in each trial, to help provide the FDA with the data it needs to make its careful determinations about the safety, tolerability, and efficacy of potential new medications for the treatment of obesity.

Back to my patient Carla at her initial visit: She is now more upbeat. She has heard of the new "GLP-1s" as she calls them and has friends who are taking them. That was what gave her enough hope to brave rush hour traffic that day to come to her clinic visit. She isn't sure the medications are right for her. She does not like the idea of a daily injection, but a weekly injection . . . maybe. She needs and wants to know more about the pros and cons of the medications as she considers them. What a great approach. There is still so much more to talk about and discuss.

7

No More New Year's Resolutions

Treating Obesity to Optimize Health

"Thank you for sharing your weight journey," I say to Yuki, a woman in her mid-forties, single and child-free by choice. Earlier, she'd shared that she was doing great in her career as a chemical engineer, but the conversation became more difficult when it turned to her weight. I tried to convey my empathy with a kind gaze. "Let's reflect and build on your past as we move forward. What are your goals? And why?"

Yuki paused for a moment, looked down at her hands, then said, "Honestly, I just want to get back into that one pair of size twelve jeans, but I feel like I should have a better goal: a health goal or some higher reason to be here, like not getting diabetes or something. But the truth is, I just want to fit into my old clothes. I want to stop spending money on new work clothes every time I gain another ten or fifteen pounds. I want to go for a jog and not chafe my thighs even though I've rubbed deodorant all over them. I want to get on a plane without worrying that I can't put the armrest down because I won't fit. I just want to feel like me."

Once a patient shares their weight journey—their struggles, their successes, the 127 ½ diets they have tried—I ask them if they have a goal. I don't say a weight goal—if that's what they share, that's okay too—I just ask if they have a goal, any goal. I want to keep the question as open-ended as possible, and for good reason: This is their chance to let me know their wishes and dreams.

Some patients don't even bring up their body. They want to travel to Costa Rica. They want to get a goldendoodle.

This *why* question is crucial. It tells me what they care about in life—and what they care about will help them stick to whatever plan we develop. Their answers will help keep them motivated as we move toward their goals: *their* goals, because it's *their* life. As a health care provider, of course I have health goals in mind for my patients. But I want to hear what motivates this one person sitting in front of me, and I want to respond to that.

Okay, so, this patient wants to get a goldendoodle. Why a fluffy dog, exactly? So I ask the question, and stay very quiet, waiting for her reply. No rush; I know it will come. And it does: She says it's because she wants to be able to go on long walks after work and play on the beach. It's because she wants to go to the dog park and make new friends. She wants to feel comfortable and have the energy to take those long outings. All this may have everything or nothing to do with her weight, but it does give me a glimpse into something this patient wants for her life.

Many people I see may feel uncomfortable, even scared of putting themselves out there like this, whether it's about dreams, life goals, or treatment. "What if the treatment doesn't work?" they think. "Isn't it better not to hope for too much?" But focusing on goals, hopes, and even dreams helps us both remember why they came in for the visit. Keeping a positive focus is important in every medical setting, but especially in treating obesity, because what we do is not about a finish line. We are focused on lifelong care, on understanding what may motivate someone to keep coming back and keep working with us. I recognize that asking for help takes courage—especially when it's not a one-and-done situation—and that the building of a relationship will be ongoing. We start with goals, and as life changes, we adjust as needed.

Care by the Numbers?

For all my soul-searching discussions with patients, there are also a lot of numbers. Specifically, tricky numbers. The numbers can be a weight on a scale, a dress size, the number of belt notches. Because while numbers are just numbers, somehow, we have attached negative meaning to them in many circumstances in medicine—especially where weight and obesity are concerned.

Even simple numbers can be laden with meaning. During my fellowship, I worked hard to say that pediatric patients with type 1 diabetes had "blood sugars within range," rather than "your blood sugars look good." What's wrong with "good" blood sugars? Well, because then there are those blood sugars that are not within range, which would translate to "bad blood sugars" and then to being ... "bad"? And why would you want to convey something so negative to a child? Or an adult, for that matter? So, this experience taught me to use the traffic light approach of red, yellow, and green foods to talk about optimal nutrition, rather than calling any given food "good" or "bad": There can be "green" and "red" foods. The leap from "I ate something bad" to "I am bad for eating that food" is just too close.

But we were talking about numbers, not Flamin' Hot Cheetos (which happened to be a red food). As I said, numbers in obesity carry a significant amount of negativity and shame for many people. For some patients, an upper threshold makes it difficult for them to feel worthy, while not crossing a low threshold makes them feel "less than." And while most of us aren't getting blood work reports every day, we can much more easily get reports for our weights. Many patients get the daily feedback of stepping on the bathroom scale. Oh, if weight were only a number, if it were only a data point, if it just gave everyone objective feedback. That would be one thing—and a lot easier to manage. But for many, seeing that number on the scale each morning is a frustrating experience in self-blame and illogic. "I went for a jog yesterday, ate small portions all day, and cooked grilled chicken, broccoli, and brown rice for dinner. Why did I gain three pounds this morning? When I went out for dinner with my friends two nights ago, there was no change in my weight. How does any of this make sense?"

It is painful to see patients who come to the research center or clinic having a number they have doggedly, relentlessly been chasing on the scale. A number that seems unattainable. Then, just when it seems within reach, it somehow slips away again—and not because of anything they have done, but because their body's biology kicks in to defend their higher body fat set point. That set point, whether they realize it or not, translates to a number that has taunted them for years, adjusting itself up, but usually not down. But most patients aren't thinking about *that* number. They just think about the three digits on the scale.

Shayna's number was 152. Just before she started nursing school, in her mid-twenties, she weighed 152 pounds, had loads of energy, and felt self-confident and beautiful. Over the last twenty-five years—during which she completed a nursing degree, raised two children, worked night shifts, and managed a busy life—she had steadily gained weight. Now she was in her early fifties, and her body wanted to hover no lower than 225 but often at 230 pounds.

At first she weighed herself daily. Then she realized that seeing the number creep up, morning after morning, was messing with her head. She was beating herself up over what—a number? How did this make sense? Her firstborn daughter was about to give birth to a child of her own. All the while Shayna was upset about these pounds ticking up on the scale when she was about to become a grandma. This was clarifying: Her *real* goal was to be the cool grandma who helped her daughter enjoy becoming a mother—by cooking for her, letting her nap, taking the baby on walks. She wanted to feel healthy for all of that.

Still, Shayna couldn't let go of the number. She was quite determined to lose at least 30 pounds to get below 200, but even at her initial visit she mentioned her goal to get to 152.

I wrote it down. If a patient has a weight number, I always note it, then do a quick BMI calculation on the NIH website calculator just to see where it falls in relation to that objective measure (again, BMI is not ideal, but it's what we have right now). Then I ask when was the last time the patient remembers seeing that number on the scale. For Shayna, it had been more than twenty years ago.

Shayna's current BMI was 37.1 kg/m^2, or in the range of class 2 obesity; her number of 152 would put her at a BMI of 24.5 kg/m^2 and would decrease her back to within "normal" range (which is a BMI of <25 kg/m^2). I do all the quick math for a few reasons: First, I want to see if the desired BMI falls within a given category (underweight, "normal" weight, overweight, obesity). I also want to give the patient a starting point and a reasonable outlook. In the past, with the older medications, Shayna's goal would have been possible but more challenging to reach and would have taken more time. With current treatments, these goals have become ever more feasible to achieve, though still with time, patience, and care. As health care providers, we always put any numbers our patients share with us within the context of health, whether they are large numbers or smaller ones. All improvements can provide health gains.

For patients who have more modest number goals, we can likely exceed them. This is a great trajectory; everyone feels awesome when they pass their benchmarks. I also have patients who get to their weight or BMI goal and then feel uncomfortable, so we ease off therapy and land where they feel more sustainably comfortable—while always presenting the pros and cons of lessening or intensifying treatment within the context of health. I start by listening to my patients' personal goals, and then we adjust and plan as we go along, depending on their health gains and how they are feeling. If they do not feel good with the current treatment plan, they are not likely to stay with it, so it's important to continuously reassess and provide guidance, including discussing benefits and potential drawbacks.

Some patients talk about goals in terms of thresholds. They say they want to get "below 150," "below 200," or "below 300." Others are less interested in body weight than weight *loss*, and have a specific number of shed pounds in mind: losing 150 pounds or 50 pounds. A few don't have a number in mind or know what health goals they are looking to attain and sometimes end up asking me, "What should my ideal weight be?" or "I just want to be healthy and feel better. What do you recommend?"

Goal Setting and Targets

Historically, because the older generations of medicine did not achieve high degrees of weight reduction, targets were not actually set, as they were much more challenging to achieve with those treatments. For decades, the most effective tool we had was bariatric surgery, which can be used for more severe obesity (for years the criteria for surgery included a BMI of ≥ 40 kg/m^2, or ≥ 35 kg/m^2 with certain obesity-related diseases; just recently the recommendations decreased to a BMI of ≥ 35 kg/m^2, or ≥ 30 kg/m^2 with certain obesity-related diseases, but insurance coverage barriers remain especially for those with a BMI of <35 kg/m^2), and some could reach their target weight depending on their starting place. But most people with obesity—about 90%—have a BMI under 40 kg/m^2 and therefore have largely relied on nonsurgical treatments.

So, what has been and is currently being used for treatment targets or goals is reaching a certain weight reduction threshold or, said another way, losing a certain percent of your total body weight. Note that this is not really a target and will likely be phased out as additional highly effective therapies are developed and we identify specific targets.

For example, many of the older medications achieved an average body-weight reduction of about 5–10%. The word "average" is important here. Patients need to know that they may not lose the average amount of weight from a trial. One person might lose 5%, while another may lose 12%, and yet another might lose 1%, or gain 1%, and so on; when the weight change is averaged for all the trial participants, it comes to 5–10%. Everybody is different. So there might be some trial and error involved in finding what is right for you.

Someone who weighed 300 pounds and took an older medication (phentermine/topiramate or naltrexone/bupropion or liraglutide) might lose 15–30 pounds, decreasing to 285 or 270 pounds. In most cases, they wanted to lose more, and a second medicine was then added to the first, and so on, until the treatment goal was met. Treatment was more challenging with fewer tools. Patients—and yes, doctors too—got exhausted or never tried treatments because of the misconception that the medicines did not work or that they would have a lot of negative side effects. There are providers, me included, who used and continue to use the older medications. Making those medicines work for patients takes dedication, time, and understanding that finding the medicine or medicine combination that targets the individual's obesity biology is possible. We do this in the context of other diseases, so we should do so for the disease of obesity. I shared an example of just such a combination therapy in my patient Swati in the previous chapter.

Today, with the new medicines like semaglutide or tirzepatide, the average weight reduction is over 15% or 20%, respectively. So, if someone has a starting weight of 300 pounds, she or he could lose on average about 45 pounds with semaglutide or 60 pounds with tirzepatide over more than a year. With percent weight reductions in this range, it becomes more feasible to discuss personal targets, because these newer medications can achieve weight reductions that are closer to if not meeting those initial goals.

For some perspective, let's look at the medical approach to some other chronic diseases. Normally, there is treatment to a specific target: for instance, for hypertension, lowering blood pressure to less than 120/80, or for diabetes we aim for a hemoglobin A1c (HbA1c) of <7% because we know specific complications are reduced below those thresholds. Percentage reduction is not used as a target for other diseases. A 10% blood pressure reduction, or a 20% decrease in hemoglobin A1c for diabetes is not how targets are chosen. So, why is it different for obesity?

Currently there are no target guidelines for obesity. It has not yet been tested if the target for optimal health outcomes is a BMI in the "normal" range (18.5–24.9 kg/m^2) or some other range. Or is the optimal BMI 22–24.9 kg/m^2? Does it matter if you are twenty years old versus eighty years old, or if you are a man or a woman, or if you are an Asian, Black, Latinx, or white person (as noted earlier, BMI is largely based on men of white European ancestry)? We do know that Asian and East Asian individuals carry more unhealthy fat per the same BMI . . . so what does that mean for choosing or adjusting goals? And remember, BMI is a screening tool, not a diagnostic measure. So it may not be great for goal setting on its own anyway.

The field is still trying to figure out the answers for what to target. For now it is likely that goal targets will be set using BMI *plus* other measures. For instance, waist circumference can help inform about the amount of belly fat. Or, better than waist circumference by itself is the waist-to-height ratio, because it accounts for body size variation. It may also make sense to combine BMI with a blood test in a similar way that the hemoglobin A1c is used for people with diabetes. It will take a lot of research to identify and validate individual or combined biomarkers for a treat-to-target strategy to become reality. We also need targets for the amount and distribution of fat mass, taking into account age, sex, and diverse populations, among other factors.

Given the heterogeneity of human obesity, target setting may require the use of a composite score where a number of variables are entered into an algorithm to estimate an individual's risk. This approach has been used successfully by incorporating factors such as age, sex, smoking history, blood pressure, and cholesterol to predict the risk of a future heart attack or other cardiovascular events within a certain time frame: If your calculated risk score is above a certain percent, you would likely benefit from additional treatment. Hopefully in the future we will be able to develop such a composite risk score for obesity. Ultimately, developing a robust, evidence-based score requires additional trial-generated, real-world, and obesity registry data, which will help us learn about health outcomes in people with obesity receiving different treatments over longer periods of time.

Whether we develop a composite score method or a biomarker, or arrive at some other eureka number down the road, this will help set guidance for health treatment goals for individuals living with obesity. There are also concerns that such numbers don't help us with:

"I want to stop trying and trying and trying—and failing."

"I want to be able to keep up with my grandkids."

"I want to be able to go into a regular store and buy 'regular' clothes."

"I want to be able to cross my legs."

"I want to feel more like me."

"I just want to feel healthier."

All of these—the *whys* of a goal—require looking at health and quality of life, not "just" pounds, inches, or notches. While numbers can help you see how far you've come, understanding your own "why" gives your progress meaning and keeps you motivated throughout treatment.

Optimizing Health

In addition to the life goals my patients set, they often come in ready to talk about their health goals: They want to feel better overall and to improve their ability to move or to join in on activities. They want to prevent obesity-related diseases like diabetes. Health also includes mental health, mood, confidence, and loving your body.

One perspective is that if you don't have to think about your health, it frees you to think about other things in your life. In this way, youth is on our side. Most twenty-year-olds do not think about back pain or aching knees or feeling crappy after staying out late with friends ... they bounce back after a hard workout, sleep in, or take an afternoon nap to rally for another big night out. Such resilience generally declines with age. Overall, aging does not give us fewer health problems; it gives us more, but maintaining or improving health generally enhances life quality. Wouldn't it be great if instead of worrying about aches and pains, you'd just be doing the things you enjoy?

"Feeling better" has a lot to do with optimizing health. Yes, weight reduction means a decrease in fat mass, and this in turn decreases the negative impacts of storing that extra fat. There are physiological changes that occur when you lose weight: Your heart doesn't need to work extra hard to get blood to the legs, arms, brain, and organs. Sleeping is more restful. Breathing gets easier. With weight loss, the pancreas no longer overproduces insulin to control our blood sugars. Losing weight is often a big step toward better health. But it's not the whole story. How we lose weight—whether it is by exercise and cutting calories or by treating obesity through recalibrating the Enough Point with surgery and medication—can also affect other health measures. There can be downsides to losing a significant amount of weight, such as loss of bone mass, muscle mass, and even hair. So, the focus really shouldn't just be on the number but on finding ways to protect and strengthen health along the way.

It is important to think about *optimizing* health, all aspects of it. Our overall health is determined by many, many factors, which can be simplified into two large buckets: nature and nurture. "Nature" includes the inherited or biological factors that influence our health. "Nurture" involves all the external or environmental factors that feed into our health and well-being. Indeed, external factors interact with our genes to determine which biologically inherited traits are expressed.

Let's say that you like living in Hong Kong. Why wouldn't you? It's an incredible city with fabulous dim sum, dragon festivals, and island hikes. But one negative about Hong Kong is the air pollution. Thick, yellow haze often clouds the city. Many people live in Hong Kong for years, their whole lives, and never develop respiratory issues like asthma or allergies. But others do.

Why is it that some get sick, and others do not? Genetic predisposition likely has a lot to do with it. Some people are just more resistant to their environment. Others may have lived there longer and been exposed to more over time. Still others may have multiple exposures; for example, a parent who smoked in the home, or a job in construction that exposed them to fumes or dust. Those earlier exposures could make them more susceptible to health problems now. Or maybe not.

Are there ways to minimize the effect of the air pollution or even prevent its impact on the lungs? In some cases, yes; in some cases, no. Some people can change jobs, but many can't without financially or professionally suffering. Most people can't just move to another place with a better air quality index. Wearing a mask may help—but for every moment of every day?

Now let's think about this same scenario in terms of obesity. Most of us live in an environment that promotes obesity. Some of us develop obesity; some of us don't. Some develop more severe obesity, some less severe. Some respond to changing their diet and adding physical activity, but once obesity develops and the brain's fat mass set point changes, therapies that target the disease mechanisms are needed. We're stuck in a metabolic Hong Kong, so to speak. (No offense to Hong Kong; it's a great city.)

We can bring in the medicines that help people lose and maintain weight and reach health goals by targeting obesity biology. But there is no medicine that directly impacts the quality of the food we eat or the motivation to exercise, or encourages other health-promoting activities. That's up to us!

If a person decides to start taking medications, it is key to pair those medications with healthful eating and physical activity. Nutritious food fuels our bodies. Exercise has health benefits that go well beyond weight maintenance: strength, muscles, bone health, mood, and the way our body uses fuel, especially glucose. We need to reimagine the goal of lifestyle changes—it's not about a number or weight. Instead, it's about optimizing health.

There are so many ways to eat healthfully. The Mediterranean diet is high in vegetables and fruits, healthy fats, and lean proteins, and can help reduce the risk of heart disease. A low glycemic index (GI) diet, which is low in foods that can spike blood sugars, is great for lowering glucose levels in people with diabetes. Physical activity has a positive impact on mood, energy, muscles—perhaps even antiaging effects. All of these health benefits are key, and yet somehow our society has prioritized size, weight, and appearance over true health and holistic well-being. Exercise has so many positive impacts; we all would benefit from decoupling the intention of weight loss from exercise. Ultimately, our bodies are the only things that allow us to live and exist in life, and being healthier allows us to live that life not only longer but better.

So yes, the medicines can reduce fat in the body. But they need to be paired with nutritious eating, physical activity, quality sleep, and stress management. The way I explain it to patients is to say, "For now, let's set aside the number on the scale—the medication(s) will help you with this; they will change the number. That number is not in your control. So, together, let's you and I focus on your health. What are the things we can think of together that you would like to and can reasonably incorporate into your life to optimize health? Let's come up with a realistic, achievable plan to do that little by little."

Oftentimes in a medical visit, we'll focus on SMART goals (specific, measurable, achievable, relevant, time-bound). For example, in one session we may pick one nutrition goal and one physical activity goal. It's best if the patient comes up with and chooses their personal goals. I listen to what a patient is sharing and help them frame it as a SMART goal.

Jerome was in his mid-fifties and eager to start a medicine to help with his weight. But he had heard from one of his colleagues that if he took the medicine without exercising, he would "get weak." In fact, his colleague shared that he'd lost over fifty-five pounds with one of the new weekly injectable medicines, which he had been happy with . . . until he went back to the gym and could not lift even half the weight he had previously been able to bench-press. He remembered his doctor talking about starting an exercise regimen when he began the medicine, but with three kids and two jobs, he had not found a way to fit in regular exercise—not until he got a new job that offered him more time flexibility. But by then he felt like he had lost a lot of muscle and was starting over.

The colleague's story prompted Jerome to commit to exercising right from the start. He had a job in IT that left him at a desk for most of the day. I asked Jerome if he had a goal in mind for adding in physical activity. He said he would work to increase exercise, but with no specifics. So I asked him what he liked doing for physical activity. He said golfing and jogging, occasionally going to the gym, and shooting hoops with his two sons in the driveway.

So, to restate his jogging as a SMART goal, we might think about it this way:

Specific—jogging (versus something you don't like to do)

Measurable—twenty minutes three times per week (versus "Whenever I can")

Achievable—three times a week (versus "Every day until I die")

Relevant—moderate physical activity (for this fifty-five-year-old
   who is already jogging once in a while, moderate intensity
   could be a goal)

Time-bound—every Saturday, Tuesday, and Thursday at 7 a.m.
   (this gets at the feasibility of "when"; if we don't plan it, it's
   really hard to do)

Then Jerome could add in two hours of golf on Sunday after-
noons, walking rather than using a golf cart. Or he could add in
twenty minutes of resistance exercise at the gym (two sets of ten
reps on five pieces of equipment) on Mondays (upper body and
abs) and Wednesdays (lower body and abs). In a few months, he
could consider switching to a standing desk.

See how SMART goals work?

Bottom line, treating obesity is not just about weight; it's actually about health, in all the ways we measure—and enjoy—it.

Shifting Your Mindset

I've seen many patients with an all-or-nothing mentality on their
weight journeys, which is so difficult to break, and yet so essential to overcome. You may feel as if there are only two ways one
can exist: eating completely healthfully (clean) or completely un-
healthfully (junk). Diet culture has perhaps contributed to this
attitude.

One of my patients, Yekta, would intermittently clean out
her entire kitchen, her entire pantry, every nook and cranny
(most often every January), getting rid of anything that was ultra-
processed or had more than five ingredients. She started doing

this once her children went off to college and she had full control of the food that came into her house. She would buy only fruits and vegetables, fish and chicken, and lean dairy. She ate "clean" for several weeks—family recipes of kebabs, mezes, stuffed eggplant— and sometimes even for several months. She would start to lose weight, but inevitably, her body would fight back, and her cravings would eventually return (as they are designed to do when living below our Enough Point). Yekta worked very hard to resist and keep them at bay. Then life would happen: Her kids would come back for an extended time, or something stressful would throw her off track, and she would go back to eating in what she called her "old way."

I think Yekta's example is more than just an all-or-none mentality. Biology drives this. When the brain's reward-motivation regions get a taste of food that they perceive to be highly satisfying, they of course want more; that's the way we're built. Taste evolved as a way to evaluate the quality, freshness, safety, and energy content of a food to ensure our bodies store enough energy. So, there is a strong subconscious incentive to seek out these highly rewarding sensations. It progressively becomes more and more difficult to consciously control every morsel of food eaten, especially since processed foods may elicit this gratification, and therefore the perceived reward potential of foods we are exposed to is very high. Eventually biology breaks through, especially if one is living below their Enough Point.

In terms of the cycle of self-blame that can accompany this situation, I am not a mental health professional, so when needed, I refer my patients to the experts. In the meantime, I advise patients to work toward increasing their awareness of an all-or-none mentality, and then, when the behavior is noticed, to start to acknowledge that we humans are imperfect and that's exactly what makes us so human. I try to arm them with the knowledge that each eating "event" is a new opportunity to fuel their body with delightful, nutritious food that can help us feel strong and healthy. And then I say, "Pick the middle one."

As an example, if confronted with a menu on which the choices are salad without dressing, breaded chicken with white pasta, and a burger with fries—how about chicken with small fries, or a burger with salad? Or how about deciding that whatever you get, you'll eat half and save the other half for lunch the next day? The point is, you don't need to be "perfect" all the time ("perfection is the enemy of good" and not realistic or attainable)—let's just pick the middle choice. The goal is not to feel deprived but rather to choose foods that fuel your body and give you energy. Additionally, it's the consistent small changes that make a difference over time, not the all-or-nothing changes that we make once in a while.

When it comes to optimizing health, consider this: If you make one positive change every month for a year, by the end of the year you will have made twelve positive changes. If you make one minuscule change every week, by the end of the year you'll have made fifty-two positive changes. *Atomic Habits*, anyone? The other thing that helped Yekta was knowing that every meal or every snack was a new opportunity for healthful eating—meaning that if she ate something she perceived to be unhealthy (let's say General Tso's chicken) for a meal, it did not mean that the entire week, or even day, was ruined. The shift to thinking about food as something nutritious and healthful, something that gives us energy and enables us to live our very best life, began to help her move away from that all-or-nothing mentality. Eating healthfully and adding physical movement will enhance your weight and health journey.

Oprah: Like others, I've found medication to be a tool—a powerful tool—that helps me manage my weight. I am so grateful for it, but I know that I need multiple tools to create a healthier life for myself. So I combine medication with hiking three to five miles a day, alternating with resistance training. If I don't have access to hiking, I use the elliptical. Or the treadmill. Or my latest and greatest favorite, the Ski-Erg, which works my arms, legs, and core. I've redefined exercise as an opportunity—a chance for me to give something back to my body so it can go a little farther. No matter what I have to give—and some days it's more than others—my goal is to move every day. Except Sunday, which I take off as a day to rest.

All this goes along with eating a healthy diet. A doctor once told me that a multipronged approach is the way it must be. She said a lot of people think they can just pick up the medication and call it done. They believe they can take it without any other counseling or lifestyle changes. But you need to be working with a health care team, coming at the issue from all different angles, the same way we treat any other chronic disease, by using every tool in your toolbox.

Another tool for optimizing health is committing to good sleep hygiene. Most of us know that we should go to bed and wake up at the same time every day—no shirking on weekends. We know it is best not to pick up our phones before bed and that we're better off if we stop drinking caffeine earlier in the day. Dark room, cool temperatures, establish a bedtime routine . . . yes, yes, and yes, if needed and possible. But what we know and what we do . . . there's a gap; we are human, not "perfect" robots. And the reality is that our world, our everyday lives, do not support even this very basic human need for sleep. In fact, a study conducted in 2013 by Dr. Rachel Markwald and colleagues found that when healthy adults were limited to just five hours of sleep per night, they burned slightly more energy—but ate even more, especially evening carbs and late-night snacks. In just a few days, participants gained nearly two pounds, highlighting how chronic sleep loss can drive weight gain. Other studies have demonstrated that the risks are even greater for night-shift workers, who face ongoing disruptions to their body clock and have higher rates of obesity, diabetes, and high blood pressure. So, disrupting or curtailing our sleep can have significant impacts on our health.

The same can be said for stress. We know that stress critically affects the Enough Point. If our life is in a constant state of stress, and this includes those everyday stressors—they simply add up. Our bodies' stress hormone (cortisol) is there to help us respond appropriately to the cold we picked up at our child's day care, to the honking horns on I-55, to the unexpected argument with a loved one, or the looming deadline at work. Stress can ramp up our appetite and trigger cravings for comfort foods. Just think of coming home after a tough day and grabbing that leftover pizza from the fridge (fat + carbs = comfort). Finding ways to manage stress, whether it's seeking supportive friends to chat with, exercising (hikes and beyond), meditating, or even pausing to take a few deep breaths in the middle of a hectic day, is an important part of optimizing health.

Ongoing Support

It is important to highlight the critical significance of mental health. I am not trained as a psychiatrist, psychologist, or therapist, so I refer patients to professionals and resources in this space. Mental health is a crucial component of comprehensive care for people living with obesity. Many have endured so much in the context of their weight. For some, the mental stress has contributed to their weight, like we saw with Julius. Some also struggle with anxiety or depression. According to a CDC report, rates of depression are as high as 40% in people with obesity; anxiety rates are estimated to be even higher. Some patients also struggle with disordered eating or eating disorders. For example, the prevalence of obesity is known to be higher in people with binge eating disorder. Support, guidance, and help from mental health professionals can be incredibly beneficial.

I discuss with my patients that prioritizing their mental health is key. If they don't have that, then no matter what goals are achieved with their weight or other medical health, quality of life may not improve. There are many psychological and psychosocial changes that occur in the setting of significant up or down weight changes. I encourage many, if not most, of my patients to work with a mental health professional while we work together on their obesity.

Though I lack a crystal ball to predict responses to the many changes that come with medical obesity treatment, guiding clues have been gathered over numerous studies and years of experience of the impact of bariatric surgery on mental health. The psychological effects from living in a very different body after losing a large amount of weight has filled many medical journals and book pages. Researchers have noted the potential for increased alcohol use and changes in relationships—including both higher divorce rates and more marriages. Some studies of patients with severe obesity who have undergone bariatric surgery have shown that the risk of self-harm may be higher following the surgery. Thus, as part of their comprehensive approach, surgeons have incorporated a mental health evaluation in preparation for and following a bariatric procedure to ensure patients get the support they need throughout their treatment.

Now that the NuSH-based medications are starting to achieve weight reduction results approaching or comparable to surgery, psychological impacts, good and bad, from losing a significant amount of weight may also likely surface. Perhaps because of social media testimonials, some patients may get the impression that these medications will fix . . . well, everything. They may believe that by treating their obesity, somehow everything else in life will fall into place. To be clear, many things do get easier—walking up the neighborhood's giant hill with your golden retriever, putting on socks, chasing after your kids, loading the car with groceries, sure . . . but life will still be life, and it won't be perfect. The rent or mortgage will still need to be paid. The washing machine will still break. Your fourteen-year-old will still disagree with you. Relationships will go well or go south. And someone's still going to have to take out the recycling.

Neither should one discount the psychological symptoms of obesity that may affect social well-being and mental health. Obesity can exacerbate feelings of loneliness or isolation, depression or anxiety. As an example, after substantial physical changes, some people still perceive themselves as being in their former body when they weighed 300 pounds, even if their current body now weighs 150 pounds. Alternatively, some people may have perceived their physical presence to be smaller when they were in a larger body, and now being in an even smaller body may be disconcerting. It can be confusing and disorienting, especially when the weight loss is relatively fast. Said another way, they know the person in the mirror has their eyes, their hair color (unless they dyed it for fun!), the same butterfly tattoo or tortoiseshell glasses, but in that glimpse they may not actually recognize the person they see.

So why is there a disconnect? When weight reduction occurs quickly—and losing a hundred pounds over one or two years is very fast—sometimes the mind's eye hasn't had time to catch up with the body's changes. Even though the weight loss may feel gradual, the change is not gradual compared to the years it took for the weight gain to occur, or the years or decades spent in their bigger body. So, when they look in the mirror, what they see on the outside may not correspond to what they see in their mind's eye.

Access to Obesity Therapies

For many, the newest, biggest source of stress isn't their body at all—it's whether they will be able to have access to the medications. Imagine shedding eighty pounds and then finding out your insurance no longer covers the treatment or that you have to change therapies or that the medication is in short supply. To face the prospect of gaining back all that weight is highly anxiety-provoking. It's no wonder some patients describe feeling a whole new layer of worry.

While these medications are transformative, unfortunately, the time of writing this book coincides with the messy middle of obesity treatment with these newer obesity medications. There is a tremendous, real need for them that has gone unmet for far too long, but health care professionals, insurers, and support systems cannot yet meet this need. In a sense, a bottleneck has occurred. In terms of health care providers, they may not be ready to prescribe these medications, as they did not learn about obesity treatments in their medical training. They may not have sufficient resources to manage the extensive, time-consuming prior-authorization process and paperwork required to obtain insurance coverage. This process is often further mired by repeated denials with ensuing appeals. There are many reasons a provider might not be ready or have the experience to guide you through a care plan with one of these medicines.

Adding to the messiness: Many patients who receive a prescription for a NuSH-based medication in the United States cannot afford them. Employer-sponsored health plan coverage is uneven and often restricted. Medicare Part D excludes drugs "when used for ... weight loss," so GLP-1-based medications aren't covered for obesity (they are covered for people with type 2 diabetes, in certain cases for people who previously had heart attacks and strokes, or for people with obstructive sleep apnea). The Treat and Reduce Obesity Act (TROA) is a bipartisan bill introduced in 2013 with the goal to improve access to comprehensive obesity care under Medicare. Medicaid coverage for obesity treatment varies by state in the US. There are ongoing discussions about how to expand coverage and decrease out-of-pocket cost for these medications in the United States given the clear health benefits demonstrated in numerous trials. As with many other medicines, the cost of GLP-1-based medications is more reasonable in some other countries, yet other countries lack commercial approval and supply of these medications.

Paying out of pocket for these medications can be prohibitively expensive. To save money and gain access to care, some turn to online platforms. Some of these platforms include highly reputable telehealth providers prescribing the FDA-approved GLP-1-based medications and older obesity medications in the context of access to a care team that may include primary care providers, endocrinologists, nurse practitioners, dietitians, and health care providers with obesity medicine expertise. They are set up to deliver comprehensive care with the important parts we just discussed (nutrition, physical activity, and more) to improve overall health. While other platforms? Not so much.

For instance, I have had people tell me that they signed up online and then simply texted their weight, height, and credit card information to that platform, and . . . voila . . . they receive a compounded substance shipped to their front door within a couple of days, if not hours. No medical telehealth visits. No medical care. Yikes! (So much for "first, do no harm.")

The GLP-1-based medications are actual medications! There is no medication that does not have risks—that is why they are available by prescription from credentialed providers with training. Their safe use requires partnership and oversight with a health care provider whose goal is to help keep you healthy and safe.

I know of some patients who have gone to a local wellness spa or aesthetics office—ones you may have passed in a strip mall with a sandwich-board sign advertising "30 Pounds of Weight

Loss in a Month!" or the like. Such venues may prescribe a compounded substance of unclear origin or composition that may not be an FDA-approved medication. The FDA and other professional organizations have issued statements warning against the use of compounded GLP-1 substances due to safety concerns. Unsuspecting people have ended up in the emergency room with severe vomiting and dehydration or worse because they received too high a dose, unsafe or unsterile research-grade material products, or something else. Reports have also suggested that people have died from use of compounded agents. Unfortunately, some purveyors of compounded products appear to be taking advantage of people's hopes of losing weight. Understandably, patients may feel desperate and want to believe this to be a viable and safe answer.

Of course, I worry about unsafe shortcuts and disreputable treatments. I also worry about the prohibitive costs of these medications limiting access to them. Given what is at stake and how long there have been no choices, many do not have the luxury to wait for costs to come down or until these highly effective medications become generic. But what is happening now is nothing short of dangerous. Dr. Jamy Ard, past president of The Obesity Society, recently said that he remains "concerned that unscrupulous actors might continue selling unregulated versions to vulnerable patients." What's happening now is not okay. My hope is, given the urgent need, the health benefits of these medications, and the potential cost savings from preventing obesity-related complications that may require interventions like dialysis or heart surgery, that we'll move through this messy middle quickly. I'm not alone in this. When I asked Dr. Donna Ryan about her thoughts, she shared: "What's exciting is that this is the beginning of real competition in the marketplace. I think we are soon going to see medications priced at less than $200 per month, and that's when payors, either insurers or out of pocket, will step up. If we are really going to impact the chronic disease burden, we must remove barriers to prescription like prior authorization and coverage denial. These powerful medications can be lifesaving, and we need to get them to those who need them."

Checking in with my patient Carla: She is fortunate that her insurance plan will pay for the medications. As we discuss her goals, she says hers is to lose eighty pounds (which for her would be about 34% body weight loss, putting her around a BMI of 26 kg/m^2), because she remembers feeling healthy and strong the last time she weighed around 156 pounds, about a year after the birth of her first son. She also wants to be able to do more. She loves dancing with her husband, but with her back and shoulder . . . then a pause and a deep breath . . . "Or truthfully, it really is my belly, Dr. Ania. I don't feel comfortable being on the dance floor with the love of my life because I am ashamed of my belly. I know he loves every bit of me, but I want to feel better, more confident, in my own body." She is also concerned that she will develop diabetes like her mother. With all this in mind, we make a plan. Given that she wants to lose nearly 35% of her body weight, unless she is a super responder to one of the highly effective medications, she may likely need more than one agent. We discuss that this goal will take some time, evaluate potential side effects, and weigh the risks and the benefits of treating or not treating her obesity. She is excited to start treatment and is hoping to see improvement in her joints, and her belly, soon so that she can enjoy dancing with her husband more fully.

8

Freedom

"It's Just as Easy to Lose Weight as It Ever Was to Gain Weight"

Oprah: When I started taking the medication, I felt, for the first time, that this is what people without obesity felt all their lives. That they do not wake up in the morning thinking, "What am I going to eat for breakfast, and is it going to be this or that?" This is what it's like to be free.

People without obesity—thin people, regular-sized people who didn't have weight as an issue—they've not been thinking about food the whole time? I felt, Wow, this frees you up to do so many other things. Look at how much brain space you have for other things. I feel more focused, more concentrated. More intensified, more vibrant. More alive. More connected. More present. All those things—because I'm not thinking about what the next meal is. I have obsessed about food my whole life, without even knowing that it was an obsession.

What am I gonna eat, and now I ate that, I shouldn't have eaten that, and oh my goodness, I didn't mean to do that, I was only gonna eat one but I ate the whole bag, and da-da-da. All of that inner voice, all of that's gone. And it's the most liberating, satisfying, redeeming feeling ever. It's just freedom. From the shackles of all the angst that food has brought into my life. I didn't know it was called "food noise" until I realized that's what was in my mind all along. And I didn't even realize how much I was shackled to it.

So many of my patients share a similar sense of amazement when they begin taking these medications. It's as if they get their first glimpse into a world that they never knew existed—and certainly had never experienced before. Food, which had consciously or subconsciously held them hostage, unsuspectingly seeping into nooks and crannies of their minds between the busyness of their lives, "like magic" (patient's words, not mine), those unrelenting thoughts of food were now no longer there. *Poof!*

Wonderfully, all that newfound space now exists for other thoughts. "Maybe I'll go swing dancing with my friends on Friday night." "I think I'll go check out that new athleisure shop that popped up on the corner." "I'm going to figure out what classes I need to take to apply for that promotion to manager at work."

Many of my patients are not consciously aware of the mental energy that fighting their higher Enough Point requires of them until it's gone. On return visits, they tell me that they're no longer drawn to the kitchen or the pantry after dinner. That sometimes they forget to eat at a "usual time" because it's not on their mind. "Forget to eat?!" they repeat. "Can you imagine?"

I can because I see it in my patients. To this day, it's still so encouraging to witness patients who are no longer mired in the intense, intrusive, persistent, disruptive food noise of their past. Their hunger occurs before a meal, not fifteen minutes after they've finished one, or, worse, waking them at 3 a.m. Cravings happen only when they smell the Sunday-morning bacon frying in the kitchen or walk by a pizzeria, not in the middle of their daughter's piano recital.

So let's talk about what to expect once someone decides to take the medications.

The Phases of Weight Change with Obesity Treatment

During the first appointment, many of my patients express hope, anticipation, and perhaps some worry, anxiety, or fear. "What if the medicine doesn't work?" they may ask. "What if I have side effects?"

"We'll take it one day at a time," I say reassuringly. "Let's talk about the side effects again, and strategies to help prevent them as much as is possible." (The next chapter, chapter 9, is devoted to side effects.)

The patient goes to the pharmacy and then home with the medicine. After taking it, some people immediately see a difference, or more accurately, they *feel* a difference—the pervasive thoughts of food begin to fade, especially if they were living well below their Enough Point. That something that almost feels like irritation or maybe anxiety that is pushing them to eat begins to fade. Others may not notice much of a change in hunger or cravings or a desire to eat. And yes, for some, the number on the scale starts to creep . . . downward. Others might not see weight loss immediately. All of this is normal—as we've discussed, every patient's experience is a little different—but in general the process includes several phases.

The Weight Reduction Phase—
Chasing the New Enough Point

When patients start responding to a medicine with weight loss, they are in the weight reduction phase of treatment. Their brain gets the signal that they have more than enough energy stores. Their body is chasing their new Enough Point, lowered by the medication. This is important, so I'm going to state it again—their body is chasing a new, lower Enough Point. Therefore, they have little interest in food and eat very little, especially in comparison to what they may have been used to eating before. Every time the dose of the medicine is further increased, their Enough Point is lowered even more, and so their body is continuing to chase a new lower Enough Point. When an additional medicine is added to an existing one (as we've commonly done with the older medications for years), their body is also chasing a new lower Enough Point. Of course, all of this is predicated on the fact that their body is responding to a particular medication. If it's not, then their Enough Point has not been recalibrated or lowered and a different medication should be tried instead.

During one of the conversations Oprah had about weight, a lively woman named Amy spoke movingly about her experience of having obesity and how the medications changed so much for her. "I was not happy in my life," she said. "My marriage was hanging on by a thread. I was in a very dark place. My world was crashing in on me. I was so ashamed of my body that I didn't like taking my kids out in public. I felt like I wasn't being a good mother. I didn't leave my house. I didn't talk to my neighbors. I had no friends. I didn't care. I was at my highest weight, about three hundred pounds. Then the inevitable happened—I was diagnosed with diabetes. My labs and blood work were scary. I remember thinking, 'This is it. This is the way I was born. This is the way I'm going to die.' I truly did not feel anything could change."

But things did change. Amy started taking a medication, and her weight dropped from 300 to 140 pounds; she was a super responder. At the lower weight, all her medical labs normalized. She said that in losing the weight, she gained so much in terms of her own health. "I took this medication and felt like I was free," she said. "I eat when I'm hungry; I stop when I'm full. It took time to adjust to this life of normalcy, but for someone like me, it's crazy to be on the other side of the spectrum where food does not control your life."

Most of what we hear on social media and in the news is about this weight reduction phase, what happens as people are chasing their new Enough Point. Most of the research that has been done has also been conducted during the weight reduction phase. We know less about the next phase, which is living in the weight plateau phase or maintenance phase in the context of treated obesity.

The Weight Plateau Phase— the New Enough Point

Every patient taking any NuSH-based medication will eventually reach a plateau—meaning they stop losing weight, plateauing at a stable weight. Oftentimes when this happens, their appetite returns, as it should, but many of my patients start to panic, thinking that the medication has stopped working. It hasn't; it's doing exactly what it is supposed to do. Let's talk about it.

Reaching a weight plateau is a very good thing. Remember the feedback loops we discussed in chapter 3 through the analogy of the thermostat? Imagine if you took a blood pressure medicine and there was no limit to how low your blood pressure would go; oh dear, that would be very unsafe. Initially you would feel dizzy, then pass out, and potentially worse. Now let's think about NuSH-based medications for the treatment of obesity. If the medicine continued to make you lose weight indefinitely, you would run out of you. You would vaporize. This is another reason why we do not call these medications weight-loss medications. Then people may think that when they stop losing weight, the medication has stopped working. But the obesity medicine is working and doing exactly what it was meant to do—keeping your weight at a new Enough Point.

At the plateau, the weight-controlling region of the brain thinks your body has enough energy, not too much or too little. At this Enough Point, energy stores are in balance, and so the appetite appropriately returns. Some days you eat a bit more, some days you eat a bit less. Your weight stays stable.

I share this with patients at the start of treatment so that they know what to expect, but oftentimes they get anxious when they reach a plateau. They might say, "I lost 40 pounds but I'm only down to 220 pounds. My goal was to get down to 180 pounds. Why isn't the medicine helping me lose more weight?" The answer is that the medicine doesn't know what your personal goal is. The medicine is just doing its job to help recalibrate and decrease your

Enough Point, but it does not "know" what your personal Enough Point goal may be. Every patient reaches their own weight plateau, determined by their individual response to a medication at a particular dose. Some patients don't plateau until they hit the weight they personally were aiming for; others plateau earlier, so we continue to increase the dose if there are higher dose steps for the medication they are taking (and they are not having side effects), or we add another medicine. We continue to do this until they reach their weight and health goals. There are also some patients who surpass their goal and we need to decrease the dose. Currently there is no way for us to predict how someone may respond to the medications, just as there is no way to know with precision how much a blood pressure medicine will decrease your blood pressure—we have a range, an average, but cannot predict your exact response beforehand. Now, why aren't we asked about this with other medicines, for example with blood pressure medicine? Well, most people don't come in saying that their goal for their blood pressure is 112/73, but people do come in with a specific goal weight of 156 pounds. Make sense?

The Weight Maintenance Phase— Living at Your New Enough Point

Once patients get to their new Enough Point, they move into the weight maintenance phase (essentially a long-term weight plateau). There are a lot of questions right now in the field about weight maintenance and a lot of questions from patients. The one I get the most often at this stage is "Can I stop taking the medication now?" followed by "I lost the weight, so I'm cured, right?"

It's important to address these common questions from the start. This sets expectations and reiterates that obesity is a chronic condition requiring continued treatment and care. Patients who have for decades assumed the personal responsibility of trying to "control" their weight find themselves thinking that it's their responsibility to sustain the lower weight (the recalibrated lowered Enough Point) that the medication enabled them to achieve. But we cannot consciously control the inner workings of our brains' Enough Point biology, no more than we can will our blood pressure to be lower by thinking about it all the time. In terms of the cure question, it may initially seem almost reflexive to think that "weight gone = problem solved," forgetting that the higher weight was a symptom of an elevated Enough Point and that now their Enough Point is being recalibrated (and maintained in this decreased state) by their ongoing obesity treatment. Weight loss does not mean a cure. For this to be a "cure," the Enough Point would have to remain at its lower setting in the absence of the medication. But a medical cure for obesity has remained elusive thus far, and this situation is not unique to obesity. As we've discussed, other chronic diseases require ongoing treatment. In the setting of diabetes, if effective medications are stopped, blood sugars rise back up. In the same way, in the setting of obesity, if effective medications are stopped, the weight is pulled back up to the previous or near previous Enough Point. Normal blood sugars in the face of active treatment do not mean the diabetes has been cured—rather it is referred to as well-controlled diabetes. "Normal" or lower weight in the setting of obesity does not mean that the obesity is cured—rather we can refer to it as well-controlled or treated obesity. This means obesity should be approached and treated as one would approach and treat any other chronic disease. If you plateau at a weight and health goal that is right for you, then you maintain that dose of the medication (or medications). If you start gaining weight, for whatever reason (e.g., in the setting of menopause, or as a side effect of another medication that causes weight gain or disease progression), then you'd work with your health care provider to discuss increasing that dose (if there are higher doses) or adding other treatment options.

Oprah: This is so crucial. I've heard Dr. Ania say this before, but I had an aha moment when we were talking on an episode of *The Oprah Podcast*. We think, "You've lost the weight—you've solved the problem." That's because in the past, every time you lost the weight, you thought, "Now this is it! I've done it! I've succeeded!" We think the problem is solved, but the problem isn't solved because the disease hasn't gone away. Just because you lost the weight doesn't mean the disease isn't still there. That is why we take these medicines. It's such an important realization.

Oprah has it spot-on. And it is an important realization—and it's also why it's so critical that we think about the words used when discussing these medications. A misconception perpetuated by word choices is that these therapies are weight-loss drugs. Coming back to this one more time, these are not "weight-loss drugs." They are medicines that target the biology of the chronic disease of obesity. Remember the definition: *Obesity is a disease where the weight-controlling regions of the brain inappropriately instruct the body to store more fat than is healthy or needed.* Obesity medications appear to be recalibrating those weight-controlling regions of the brain so that we store less fat. Reducing the extra fat tissue is one way to improve our overall health. Recalibration of that Enough Point with medications does not "fix it" at that level. The distinction matters in our understanding of what obesity is and how to treat it.

Patients aren't the only ones with questions: Health care providers are considering whether patients can be switched to other medications (usually because of lack of access to medicines, current high cost, or lack of insurance coverage for the medications). Right now, if financially feasible, patients stay on the medicine or medicines that helped them recalibrate their Enough Point and lose weight to reach a new (lower) Enough Point. This is no different from what we do when treating other chronic diseases. If a particular medicine (for example an ACE inhibitor or beta-blocker for treating elevated blood pressure) helped a patient normalize their blood pressure, then we would continue that medicine at the dose that worked for them. If the obesity medications were covered by insurance and did not have a high out-of-pocket cost, we might not be asking ourselves these questions about stopping to such an extent. Currently, there are many questions about "maintenance therapy" and potentially switching patients to different medications once they reach the weight maintenance phase—perhaps the patient can switch to a medicine with less frequent dosing or an oral formulation. Studies are ongoing to address these and many more questions about the weight maintenance phase. More to come!

And what if weight gain begins to occur in the weight maintenance phase? One issue is we do not currently know if this is weight regain or disease progression. And how do we best maintain the weight loss and the health improvements that have previously been gained? More work is needed to better understand this, but for now we increase the dose or add a medicine.

Health Benefits

An astounding transformation has been taking place within the last few years. Study after human study has demonstrated that treating obesity improves health beyond just weight reduction and substantially improves outcomes for obesity-related complications such as heart disease, diabetes, kidney disease, fatty liver disease, heart failure, obstructive sleep apnea, and knee osteoarthritis. Treatment with the new medications also fairly consistently improves blood pressure and cholesterol levels. Now it almost seems like "Well, of course it does," but during those years when treating obesity was unfortunately seen as a cosmetic issue, studies were required to prove the clear health benefits of treating obesity. Good news: We now have these studies, and more are coming!

A few pivotal studies are important to highlight. One that stands out focused on heart health—and was the first study of its kind in participants with obesity but without diabetes. Leading up to this study, there were many studies looking at heart health in people with diabetes (but not in those with obesity alone). The studies were initially designed to prove that the GLP-1-based medications were not harmful to patients with diabetes—specifically that they did not increase cardiovascular events (such as heart attacks and strokes). What emerged from these studies was that not only were the medications not harmful, they were actually helpful for heart health in people with diabetes.

Enter the SELECT cardiovascular outcomes trial, which included over seventeen thousand people with obesity (but without diabetes) who previously had a heart attack or stroke. Participants were randomized to receive semaglutide versus placebo for up to five years. The study was massive, took years of planning, and almost didn't happen given its size and expense. I served as a site investigator for this large global trial. The trial drew to a close in 2023, and the results were quickly prepared for the publication. The excitement was palpable in the standing-room-only convention center space at the American Heart Association's (AHA) Scientific Sessions on a cool November day in Philadelphia. Dr. Michael Lincoff, from the Cleveland Clinic, presented the primary results to an eager crowd of cardiologists with co-chair Dr. Donna Ryan in the audience. I had been asked to be the discussant—the person who gives their expert opinion on the study design and the results. In essence, I was given just seven minutes to convey to thousands of cardiologists that treating obesity was critical in treating heart disease. My message was simple and captured in the title of my talk: "When Treating Cardiovascular Disease . . . SELECT Treating Obesity." The data spoke for itself: Was there a clear benefit observed in preventing a second heart attack or stroke by treating patients with obesity with semaglutide? The answer was a resounding yes! What about people with obesity who have not previously had a heart attack or stroke? The SURMOUNT-MMO trial is now ongoing to see if tirzepatide can prevent a first heart attack or stroke in those who are at high risk or if it can prevent a second heart attack or stroke in those who have previously experienced such an event. Many other trials are now ongoing with medications that are not yet approved for obesity treatment to see if those also improve heart health. The SELECT trial was the first of its kind in the obesity space; it was pivotal. This trial led to the FDA's approval of semaglutide for the prevention of repeat heart attack or stroke in adults with obesity and established cardiovascular disease.

Several other important studies have recently been completed demonstrating the benefits of semaglutide and tirzepatide for patients who have heart failure with preserved ejection fraction (HFpEF, a condition where the heart is able to pump but does not fill effectively), significantly improving various measures of quality of life (STEP-HFpEF and SUMMIT). A study with tirzepatide demonstrated clear improvements in sleep apnea (treated with and without CPAP, continuous positive airway pressure) in the context of significant weight reduction (SURMOUNT-OSA). This trial led to the FDA's approval of tirzepatide as the first medication indicated for the treatment of sleep apnea. Several studies with semaglutide or tirzepatide exhibited improvements in fatty liver, kidney disease, knee osteoarthritis, and the list goes on and is anticipated to increase with many more ongoing studies. This is all key because treating obesity is about improving health, and so far what we have seen in these NuSH-based medication trials points to just that: These medicines are clearly improving health by effectively treating obesity.

Of course, as these medications, including semaglutide and tirzepatide, were initially developed and FDA approved for the treatment of diabetes, there is no debate that they all improve diabetes outcomes. But, as we discussed in chapter 5, a key finding in these trials is that participants who already have diabetes lose less weight with these medications than those who have obesity but do not (yet) have diabetes. Trials with both semaglutide and tirzepatide, as well as older medications, demonstrate this phenomenon. These data points provide yet another reason not to wait to start treatment until obesity progresses to full-blown diabetes (or any other obesity-related disease, for that matter). Treating obesity early, before obesity-related complications develop, may provide a window of opportunity to have the greatest impact on health outcomes. This is echoed especially in children and adolescents who may develop obesity-related diseases even during childhood.

Sawyer was just thirteen years old when, during a follow-up visit for his childhood obesity and prediabetes, his blood sugar level was checked and was found to be high. His A1c was checked on the spot, confirming his new diagnosis of type 2 diabetes. Over the next few months, his doctor started him on treatment with metformin and a NuSH-based therapy for his obesity. His weight came down and his blood sugars improved without any additional medications. Since then his diabetes has been well controlled and essentially remains in remission. One of the most important takeaways is that when we're treating obesity, we're helping people lead healthier, hopefully better-quality, lives. For Sawyer, his life and health trajectory were changed immeasurably with his early treatment. As my Yale pediatric endocrinology colleague Dr. Michelle Van Name shares, she is "eager for a future in which children and their families are not faced with needing to manage obesity-related conditions in their teens and as young adults because they have benefitted from options for an early, comprehensive, and health-focused treatment approach."

Additionally, exciting studies are investigating whether these medications can actually *prevent* obesity-related diseases. For example, if the medication was taken before the patient had type 2 diabetes, could it prevent diabetes?

I led a recent study, which was a continuation of the SURMOUNT-1 trial with tirzepatide, in which we focused on treating people with prediabetes. Because all the study participants in this second part of the trial had prediabetes, they were at higher risk for heart disease, stroke, and kidney disease and had a 25–70% higher chance of developing type 2 diabetes over the next five years. Fortunately, the study outcome found that, as long as they took tirzepatide, the risk of developing diabetes was decreased by 94%, and that nearly 99% of the participants did not progress to diabetes over the three years of the trial. These results established that type 2 diabetes could be delayed or prevented by starting obesity treatment early in those who are already at increased risk. The implications of this are remarkable. Nearly a hundred million people have prediabetes in the United States, and even if one in three of these individuals develops diabetes over the next five years, that's an additional thirty million people with diabetes— add this to the nearly forty million people who are already living with diabetes in the United States. Diabetes is a leading cause of blindness, kidney failure, and many other downstream diseases. With these medications, we could potentially prevent progression from prediabetes to diabetes and improve the long-term health of tens of millions of people.

Other Benefits

Some of my patients marvel at other quality-of-life enhancements. Take Lynn, who's in her thirties, with a bubbly, positive personality, the high half-bun, half-ponytail atop her head bobbing as she rapidly chats with me. She's single, with a close-knit family, and, in her words, a "doggie momma" to Mimi, her Shih Tzu. When I first met Lynn, she had severe obesity, with a BMI of >50 kg/m^2 and a weight over three hundred pounds. At that time, so many things in her life that should have been enjoyable just weren't.

She described a trip to the beach when she was at her heaviest. "I felt so uncomfortable," she explained. "Two summers ago, I could barely make it up the stairs. Walking on the beach was torture. I broke my chair—it was rusty, but still, I broke it. And the fatigue. Just getting in and out of the chair—it would take an act of God to get me out of that chair."

Lynn has since lost over one hundred pounds. She told me what it's now like to go to the beach. "I still had some difficulty with a low chair," she said. "But now I can get up out of that chair. I was walking on the beach, enjoying it like I did when I was a kid—just like any other person." I'm so happy for Lynn and all my patients who feel their lives are more free, to travel with family and enjoy places that they love. Even just simple things like taking a stroll on the beach.

Simple Pleasures

Oprah's producer Brian shared his heartfelt story about taking the new medications on one of the episodes of *The Oprah Podcast* that we taped about obesity treatment with the new medications. He spoke about how, as he lost weight, he finally felt seen and wanted to be seen. When I spoke to him later, he reminded me of something else I hear from many of my patients. "I purposely did not look in a mirror for probably fifteen or twenty years," he told me. "I avoided *all* mirrors. I was up to a 3- or 4XL." But now he says he feels fine about how he looks—even with what he calls his "turkey wattle" and loose skin. "I'm solidly at an XL," he says. "Now my husband and I can go shopping together, and that's a joy. It is a joy knowing you could walk into a store and just . . . buy clothes."

It sounds so simple, doesn't it? But for my patients, not having to go to a special store or scroll endlessly online to find clothes that are made for their size, and instead walking into a store, is such a source of delight and freedom.

Another benefit my patient Alice noticed right away was that her knees stopped hurting. She woke up one morning without knee pain. It was just like that. What a thrilling change! She no longer had to plan out her activities based on when she thought her knees would give out. She simply did all the things she needed to do.

This was not just a one-off. Another patient, Tonya, a local farmer in her forties, did not realize that she had joint pain until it disappeared. She just assumed the achiness was part of getting older—nothing to do but get on with it. When she started taking the medications, suddenly the pain went away. What a surprise. Was this a fluke? No, not for her it wasn't. When she temporarily stopped taking the medications because of the shortage, the pain returned before the weight did.

In both Alice's and Tonya's cases, the relief may potentially be in part due to diminishing the inflammation that may have contributed to the pain. Obesity and inflammation are intimately intertwined, so treating obesity can help alleviate inflammation. Decreasing the amount of weight any joint bears will also help protect it from the gravitational stress of carrying extra weight, but what was interesting at least in these two patients was that both women noted the relief happened *before* significant weight loss. This phenomenon needs to be investigated further through physiology studies to understand the potential mechanisms that may be leading to such benefits.

How Others React to Weight Loss

I could tell many stories that my patients share with me about how they are able to live life with more ease and more enjoyment, more freedom, but I would be remiss if I didn't also mention some of the changes that they didn't anticipate that are not all positive.

For example, my patient James started taking a medication during the pandemic. When he walked into the conference room after the return to the office, no one recognized him. That is, until he started speaking. This man sounded like James. His blue eyes looked like James's, but they were now outlined with gray-rimmed glasses. His face was shaved and smooth, whereas previously James had a goatee. The other, major thing that was confusing everyone: This person was half James's size.

As it turned out, James had developed type 2 diabetes during lockdown and began a highly effective weekly injectable medicine, which he had paired with a healthier diet, focusing mainly on decreasing sugar and cutting out as much highly processed food as possible. Additionally, to relieve the anxiety he felt during the pandemic, he started to exercise, to walk and then jog, which eventually led him to train for a 5K race.

Over about a year and a half, he had lost more than a third of his body weight, over ninety pounds. The transformation was remarkable.

James was, of course, exactly who he had always been. Yes, he'd experienced his changes somewhat in isolation. There was no requirement at his job to keep the Zoom camera on during calls, and James had kept his camera off. No one from his job had witnessed the day-by-day progression as the pounds came off and his strength grew. James himself was still adjusting to his new body—in a lot of ways, it had happened very quickly. In some respects, he could not remember what it was like to live in a large body, but in other ways he was still the twelve-year-old boy being bullied on the playground for his weight.

Everyone at the marketing firm began to comment about James's new appearance:

"What did you do?"

"You look fantastic!"

"You must feel so great!"

"I *gained* thirty pounds during the pandemic. How did you lose all this weight?"

Was any of this questioning fair to James? Did he want to talk about his obesity? No one said anything about his diabetes—no one could *see* his diabetes—but everyone had something to say about his weight. These conversations took James by surprise.

Everyone Knows . . .

James's experience reminds us that obesity is a visible disease, and the impact of treating obesity is . . . also visible. While diseases like vitiligo or cystic acne are visible, other diseases like high blood pressure and high cholesterol are not obvious, and we can choose to share or not share treatment or whether we are worse off or improving. No one can eyeball your cholesterol or tell from a glance that your blood pressure is off the charts.

But with obesity, *everyone* knows. And there are people out there—strangers, even—who feel it's absolutely fine to comment on it. Suddenly, everyone becomes an expert on weight. They may offer encouragement, cheerleading, or camaraderie. Sometimes they may be discouraging, jealous, or even try to sabotage efforts.

Some relationships might become stronger; some weaker. Some married patients will get divorced; others will grow in the relationship with their partner. Some will find that a few of their friends are jealous, while other friends feel joy in seeing them move through this journey. It's often a mix of responses, and oftentimes difficult to predict. This is where shame can emerge again. Our patients are shamed if they take the medications—"You took the easy way out." They are shamed if they don't take the medicine—"Why don't you do something about your weight?" They are shamed if they don't lose weight, and they are shamed if they do lose weight.

On one of the episodes we taped for *The Oprah Podcast*, we heard the perspective of Michaela, who lost 165 pounds over two and a half years through bariatric surgery and, after that, one of the new medications. "I wish I could say, 'Oh my gosh, it's just been the most perfect experience ever,' but I've truly been [cycling] through these three emotions, and it's been happy, sad, and mad," she told us. "I'm happy because I'm finally who I've always wanted to be, and I finally got the help that I needed.... I'm also sad, I'm very sad, because no one would listen to me—I was constantly blamed for such a long time. I think about the life I could have lived if somebody would have helped me. Then anger because ... I constantly get told, 'Oh, you're so pretty.' 'You're such a nice person.'" A part of her wants to ask them why they're saying these things *now*, "because I've always been Michaela."

She also admits not everyone in her life has been supportive. "When you say you're going to lose all this weight," she says, "people automatically assume it's because you hated yourself, and that's not the case for me. I love myself so much that I wanted to make this change." Oprah stopped her and said, "That's *huge*. . . . That's powerful." It is so important.

Michaela assumed that the people who cared for her would support her weight journey. "What I've noticed is: A lot of the people that would invite me to things and that would show up for me stopped," she says. "I'm not sure if they enjoyed me more as the background friend. . . . I would have probably been dressed in all black trying to mute myself out, and for no one to see me. Now I love to be seen. I love to talk and to be the center of attention in these types of situations. And I have to ask myself, 'Did they prefer me the way that I once was before?'"

My patient Lynn, whom we met earlier in this chapter, echoed this disorientation. She described having obesity as having armor. She knew that the people who cared about her and truly loved her did so regardless of what size she was. Now, with new attention, including romantic interest from men, she felt like she didn't necessarily know if they liked her for who she was or if they were drawn to her for what she looked like.

That said, she recognized that the way she interacted with the world was very different after her weight loss. So she wondered, how much was them . . . and how much of the change was due to her?

She said, "I definitely think my energy is more positive. I can feel it. I was kind of not speaking with my neighbors, like standoffish with them, and now they all just want to approach me and talk to me, and they tell me how good I look when I'm walking Mimi. I'm putting out better energy for sure. As opposed to an anxious, scared, fearful energy."

Lynn also described interactions with the people who know her well. She has one set of friends who won't bring up her weight at all. They've not once mentioned the fact that she has lost 115 pounds since starting to take a medication. She also has a set of friends from college who have always been very supportive of her, at every size.

Lynn recently got together with one of these college friends again—the first time she'd seen her since she'd lost over a hundred pounds. After spending the day together, Lynn's friend said to her, "You look great! How do you feel?" Lynn explained what that question meant to her: "It was such a nice moment for me, because she hadn't seen me in a while, and I knew she loved me. I put in all this hard work, and it paid off. It just felt so good. We walked around and I did not get winded. We enjoyed that simple day. I don't think she realizes . . . how important it was to me. I felt I could conquer the world. I still have obesity, but I can be joyful."

I think that's such a powerful story—and such a good example of how everyone can support people with obesity. It reminded me of another conversation from one of the *Oprah Podcast* episodes we taped, when we spoke to Jewel, a young woman who'd shared her story of losing 107 pounds, thanks to the new medications. She and her mother had met Oprah before this podcast taping. At that time, it was clear her mother, Marissa, wasn't comfortable with having her daughter on an obesity medication. Oprah says she noticed the moment during the conversation that Marissa realized that obesity is a disease—one that can be treated. On the podcast, she asked Marissa if learning that fact had shifted her opinion of the medications. "Absolutely," Marissa said. "It really has been a game-changer. And I've been kind of like a champion for other parents who have those same questions. I'm just like . . . 'Check the root of your resistance—and understand [your child's] experience.' I've never thought about going to the theater and worrying about the seat in the theater. Or that you can't sit in the exit row. We're tall and have long legs, and we prefer the exit row. That wasn't an option for her. I didn't know that there were policies for extra seats [that those with obesity must purchase]." Marissa realized that she did not fully understand her child's experience in the world, even though she and her daughter have a very close relationship. "I really had to educate my ignorance," she said on the podcast. It was wonderful to see Marissa's shift in opinion—from reluctance to fierce support—and to see Jewel smile and nod as her mother spoke.

Takeaways

What many of my patients learn is that there could be a million reasons why other people choose to share an opinion about their weight loss. Maybe it's a comment made with the best of intentions—they are somehow trying to relate. Or maybe it's their way of attempting to understand why and how such a significant change occurred. Or maybe in some instances, it is judgment. Or maybe it's a reflection of their own insecurity and discomfort.

The feedback might be small—how much eye contact someone makes. Or it might be more significant, as Lynn and Michaela found with some of their friends stepping back. Or as James realized, it might be the presence or absence of unrequested feedback.

He used to hear things like: "I see you have salad for lunch, James; great to see you making those healthy choices!" or "We're running a 10K fundraiser race this weekend, but you probably can't join us for that." Those sorts of slights were gone—that was a good thing.

With these shifting relationships, communication—finding new connections while fostering ongoing support—is key. I've seen, among my patients, that everything can change, from who does the grocery shopping and cooking to what's for dinner to all of a sudden having a love of biking or weight lifting or painting. Activities and interests can change, energy levels can change, eating habits can impact seemingly simple activities like going to dinner. New threads can emerge, in terms of a change in the power dynamic between people, such as feelings of insecurity or even jealousy. As mentioned, you may need guidance from a mental health professional to help navigate relationships.

While the interpersonal dynamics in my patients' lives may change in rewarding ways, the most important relationship is the one they have with themselves. Michaela, who circulated between feelings of happiness, sadness, and anger, says she always falls back to happy. "I'm just happy I'm here now," she says. "I'm happy I'm able to tell this story and advocate for other people just like me."

As I continue my conversation with my patient Carla, she brings up again that her mother, her sister, her uncle, and her grandparents all had diabetes. Such family history, and thus genetics, significantly increases the likelihood that she will also develop diabetes, especially considering her obesity. Her mother also had breast cancer in her sixties and her sister had been treated for endometrial cancer. Carla's physical exam reveals a borderline increase in blood pressure, acanthosis nigricans in the armpits and back of the neck (a type of darkening and thickening of the skin associated with prediabetes), and an office hemoglobin A1c of 6.3% (6.5% or greater is diagnostic of diabetes). A physical exam of her thyroid and liver is normal. She doesn't have deep-red-colored stretch marks on her belly but instead pale-colored ones, steering away from the very rare diagnosis of Cushing's syndrome. She is strong and does not have any muscle weakness, also a reassuring marker of the absence of additional disease. Her history, review of medications, blood work, and other parts of her physical exam suggest that there are not any other underlying or contributing causes to her obesity (such as medications that promote weight gain). Though at increased risk for obesity-related complications, she has a great primary care provider and is up-to-date on her preventative health screening.

That said, I am quite concerned about her risk of progressing from prediabetes to diabetes. In addition to the many benefits of treating her obesity, based on clinical studies of participants who closely resembled Carla, we can predict with a degree of confidence that at least for the next several years, with treatment, we can help prevent her from developing diabetes. I explain all that I had seen that was reassuring and also shared my concern with Carla. She listens, and we consider next steps.

9

Let's Get Real

Side Effects of the Medications

Unfortunately, there is no medicine for any disease that does not have any side effects. Insulin can cause blood sugars to drop down to dangerously low levels. Birth control pills can cause melasma (brown or hyperpigmented patches on the face). Sildenafil (Viagra) can cause headaches and blue vision (yes, you read that right).

Obesity medications are no different. When I see a new patient, often their biggest fears are about the potential side effects. They may have seen TikTok videos of people who are taking these medications and experiencing nausea or vomiting. Others mention a friend or family member who was prescribed one of the new medications by their health care provider and lost a lot of weight quickly but endured a lot of side effects.

I understand these concerns—they are valid. No one wants to experience side effects to any medicine for any disease.

You or someone you know may be in this very place of indecision about the medicine right now, with questions such as: "Will I feel nauseated?" or "I hate vomiting—do I really want to risk it?" or "I heard that some people have diarrhea or constipation—there is no private bathroom at work. How will I manage?"

Let's start with the most common side effects of the GLP-1-based medications, which are the gastrointestinal side effects, namely: nausea, diarrhea, constipation, and vomiting. There are several things to know about these common side effects. First, they most often occur as the dose of the medicine is increased or if the medicine dose is increased too quickly. So if the dose increases are slowed down, these side effects can be mitigated if not wholly prevented. Second, these side effects usually subside once the dose of medicine has been unchanged for some time. Third, if these side effects occur, they are usually mild, sometimes moderate, but generally not severe. And finally, although these are the most common side effects, they do not occur in everyone.

We can look to the clinical trials of the once-weekly injectable medications to better understand how people may be affected. It is important to consider, though, that there is a lot less flexibility in dose increases or adjustment in clinical trials with participants than in clinical practice with patients. This is because in a study, we need to follow a protocol, or a set of procedures, so that we know each participant is receiving treatment as intended. So if the protocol says we need to increase the dose after four weeks, then that's what we need to do; we cannot slow down the dose escalation unless the protocol allows for that. More recent trial protocols allow for more flexibility with dose increases to help mitigate the potential side effects.

Overall, trials are standardized with rigorous procedures to get the clearest assessment of a medicine—is it safe, what are the side effects, how well does it work? The FDA requires at least one year (fifty-two weeks) of patient data on a given treatment dose for these NuSH-based medications. So the studies are designed in such a way that participants quickly reach the treatment doses over a prespecified period of time and then remain at those doses for at least one year. The dose escalation rate (stepping up of the medicine dose from low to high) that is used in the trial is then included in the FDA package insert for the medication. It is not uncommon for a provider to institute this dose escalation rate into their clinical practice as that's what has been studied in the trials. That said, there is no requirement to increase the dose as quickly as is done in trials. By rapidly recalibrating and lowering the Enough Point again and again (with each step up in dosage), speedy dose escalation increases the prevalence and severity of side effects. With the Enough Point lowered too quickly, it may feel like you've eaten a full Thanksgiving meal at breakfast, another one at lunch, and then another one at dinner, even though you may have eaten much less than what you are accustomed to eating. The brain is screaming "Enough!"

Outside of a trial setting, in clinical practice, a strategy that considers an individual's tolerance of dose increases may reduce some, if not most, of the gastrointestinal side effects. For example, if a treatment is prescribed and the patient is experiencing nausea relating to the medication, waiting until the nausea has resolved for several weeks on that initial dose may help decrease the severity of nausea if the patient requires the next higher dose to reach treatment goals. If side effects continue or are significant, the dose can be decreased. In general, the medications become more tolerable over time, so dose increases can be slowed down until the patient's side effects subside.

The rates of common gastrointestinal side effects observed in participants in later-stage (phase 3) clinical trials of once-weekly medicines that are already FDA approved may help better set expectations. Still, there is the caveat that the trial doses for the study participant may be increased more quickly than what would work best for the individual patient in clinical practice.

In the trials, nausea has been the most commonly reported side effect with the family of GLP-1-based medications. Notably, this is also the case for the placebo group. In the arms of the trials that receive the highest dose of the medications, 30–45% of participants report the occurrence of nausea at least once if not more often during the course of the trials, which typically last more than a year. If a trial participant develops nausea, it is most likely to occur near the beginning of the trial, when the study medication doses are being increased. The occurrence of nausea generally tapers once the dose of the medicine levels out.

You may be asking yourself: But why does nausea occur in the placebo group, albeit at a lower rate, and in a similar time pattern as the treatment group? One potential explanation is that although participants are blinded as to whether they are getting active medication or placebo (as are the investigators), they know to look out for these side effects. Another possibility is that since some participants joined in the trial for a chance to receive treatment for their obesity, they may actually hope to have some side effects as a sign that they are getting the study medication. Participants are people living in the real world—during the year or more of the trial they, too, can get carsick or eat too much of Uncle Jason's brisket. Though rare, there are occasional patients for whom the side effects persist, and this is an important consideration in clinical practice and underscores the need to develop additional therapeutic tools targeting different mechanisms.

Constipation or diarrhea occurs in about one in four people in the medication groups of the trials. Both tend to be more frequent during the dose escalation period, but constipation is more likely to persist over time in some participants.

In the arms of the trials that receive the higher doses of the GLP-1-based medications, vomiting is reported in 10–20% of participants at least one or more times over the course of the year or more; lower doses have lower rates of vomiting. Like with nausea, vomiting also occurs in the placebo group, just certainly at lower rates. Why would someone in the placebo group have vomiting—stomach bug? There are also other medications (which both the medication and placebo groups may be taking) that cause nausea and sometimes vomiting: these include certain antibiotics, ibuprofen, certain blood pressure medications, opioids, and certain antidepressants. Bottom line, these participants are living their lives in the real world.

For the higher-dose groups in the trials, one in five is still a lot to have any vomiting, even if it occurs only a few times. That's why with patients in my clinic, we go up on the doses slowly. If someone is having nausea, we do not go up on the dose, and sometimes we even go down on the dose—we want to prevent any vomiting, and most often we do.

The GLP-1-based medications have been used for over twenty years in patients with type 2 diabetes, and interestingly, their reported rates of these side effects, including nausea and vomiting, are lower in the trials; we don't know why this may be the case. As newer medications are being developed, researchers are looking for ways to have fewer side effects and less need for slow dose changes.

In the future, it is likely we'll have medicines that are even more tolerable. For now, let's talk about potential ways you and your provider can work together to mitigate or prevent side effects.

Start Low, Go Slow

A great way that your provider can help you prevent or limit side effects is by starting low and going slow. What does that mean? Well, let's begin with "start low." It is important to start at the lowest available dose of the medicine. This applies to anyone who is first starting these medications or anyone who has paused treatment for any reason.

Let's say you start taking a medication and you do not have any side effects with the once-weekly injection. After a month, if your goals indicate that more weight reduction and additional health benefits are needed, your provider can consider increasing the dose. But if you experience nausea and after a month you're still having it, then likely the same dose would either be decreased if it is intolerable or would be continued until your body gets used to the medicine. If you're having nausea with some vomiting, your provider may likely decrease the dose. If the medicine comes as a single-dose injector device without the possibility of a lower dose, then, as a work-around, your provider may recommend that you take it less frequently than once a week. If instead the medicine comes in a multi-dose pen where each click of the pen increases or decreases the dose by a very small amount, then your provider may have you take fewer clicks as a way to receive a smaller (micro) dose and may recommend a much slower dose increase over a longer period of time. It is essential for all of this to be done under supervision of a medical provider. Obesity medications have both intended beneficial effects and side effects, just like any other medication.

There are additional strategies that your provider may recommend to avoid gastrointestinal side effects like diarrhea or constipation. For example, increasing water and/or fiber intake or adding stool softeners for constipation.

Some additional strategies your provider may recommend to decrease gastrointestinal side effects include:

- Avoiding eating past the point of fullness. For example, eating more slowly or pausing for a few minutes before getting up for meal seconds. Things you may find helpful are not serving the food in the middle of the table (family-style), where it is easy to reflexively and quickly refill, and instead serving food from platters on the counter or stove. These will give time for your brain's fat-mass-regulating regions to kick in and help prevent eating beyond your new Enough Point.

- Noting which foods exacerbate your side effects. Because certain foods may cause more side effects than others, keeping a diary of foods and symptoms may be helpful, especially when starting a new medication. This aids in identifying which foods may cause you to have side effects so that you can potentially reduce them, especially during the time the dose of the medication is being increased. For some, fatty foods cause the most side effects; for others, spicy foods or carbonated beverages. It's not that these foods cannot be eaten ever again—it's just that during the weight reduction phase you will likely want to eat less of them. Don't worry, your favorite chocolate-chip ice cream could become your Friday-evening treat again once your weight plateaus—albeit in smaller amounts. During the active weight reduction phase, you may be completely satisfied by one or two bites of the creamy deliciousness. It's important to work with your provider and be patient with the process. For some it becomes an opportunity to delve into healthful eating now that the food noise, intrusive cravings, and insistent hunger have abated.

- Eating more frequently, but in lesser amounts. You might find eating small amounts throughout the day (cottage cheese with cherry tomatoes in the morning, an apple with a piece of string cheese for a mid-morning snack, and so on), rather than sitting down for several big meals, works better for you. Patients who eat one large meal while starting to take these medications may experience more side effects. If you are a woman who has been pregnant at some point in your life, you may remember having to break up your meals into smaller quantities. Remember those six to ten almonds that were meant to be your snack and you thought were ridiculous? Well, now you may find that serving size to be perfectly reasonable as you're losing weight.

- Make sure to stay well hydrated. You may find that you are less thirsty in addition to less hungry. Food contains water. When you eat less, you will take in less water. You may feel more nauseated when you are dehydrated, and drinking water can help. So remember to fill your water bottle first thing in the morning and set goals throughout the day—your kidneys will thank you!

- Finally, let your provider know if you are having any side effects. They are there to help you! It's important to let them know early so that side effects can be mitigated rather than get worse.

Gastrointestinal side effects are most likely to peak between days one and three after the injections and coincide with the biggest increase in the medication in your body. So eating less or lighter foods on those days may also be helpful. Knowing when peak symptoms occur for you helps to determine what day of the week to take your medication. Some people choose to take their medications on Sunday evening. They're usually those who do not want to have side effects on the weekends (the party crew! the weekend warriors!). If they have side effects, the peak would then occur sometime between Monday and Wednesday. Patients who take the medicine on Fridays, on the other hand, don't want to have any side effects while at work (hello, worker bees!). They prefer to be at home during the weekend if they are to have side effects from a dose increase.

Esther's Story

When I first saw Esther, she was in her seventies, a retired postal worker, a breast cancer survivor, and newly in love with a wonderful partner and travel companion. She was highly motivated to treat her obesity, and this goal was stronger now, given her newfound love. She wanted to maximize the number of healthy and happy years they would have together. She had previously tried some of the older medications, which worked to a small extent but didn't give her the health gains that she was looking for. She also experienced side effects that made her reluctant to continue.

When the new medications became available, she had also tried them, but the side effects were unbearable, so she made an appointment to see me. We decided to start very slowly, using extremely low doses (with a multi-dose injector pen). Every week she would increase her dose by just two clicks (so it took many weeks to get to the initial dose of the medication). If at any point the nausea returned, she remained on the current dose until the symptoms abated.

Esther had been ready to give up hope, but within several months, she was able to increase her dose to one where she had a consistent weight reduction without nausea or vomiting. It took a long time and a lot of patience, but she reached her weight and health goals of losing about twenty-five pounds over just a year, and her blood pressure improved during that time as well. It just took some listening, support, and patience. And not giving up.

Missed Doses

Another important point to remember if you are taking a weekly injectable obesity medicine is that if you are not on the starting dose of the medication and miss more than two injections in a row (so more than two weeks), you may likely need to restart the medication at a lower dose to give your body time to readjust. Restarting at the higher dose may be a jolt to your system even if you did not have side effects previously. After a few weeks, the medicine is mostly out of your system, so your body forgets that it got used to it. It needs the reminder by slowly restarting.

Think of it this way: Because of how long they last, the medications build up in your body over time. While the peak levels in the body are within the first few days, by the end of the week the levels have decreased by about half. (This is a lot longer than many of the medications that we take by mouth daily: In that case half the drug is gone after a few hours or within a day—hence the need to take those oral medications daily.) Then the second weekly injection is added to the remaining half dose from the first injection. With the third injection, it is added to the remainder from the second injection plus the tail end of the first injection (which is about a quarter of the initial peak). By the fourth week of a specific dose, the medicine in your system starts to reach the "steady state" level. That is why it takes at minimum one month (at least four injections) before your provider may advance you to the next dose of a weekly injectable medication. The weekly injectable medications take nearly four weeks to get to a steady state in your body.

As long as there are no side effects and weight is not lost too quickly (no more than 1% per week of your body weight is a good rule of thumb), then after four weekly injections, and following a discussion with your provider, it may be time to increase the dose. But if you are losing weight, even just a little bit, it is more than okay to wait before increasing the dose of medicine, and indeed this may very well be what your provider will recommend. You may not need a higher dose of medication. Many may choose to stick with the dose they are on until their weight plateaus as a way to minimize the chance of side effects while also seeing the outcome of the medicine on their weight and other health measures. Once the weight levels off, your health care provider may recommend increasing the dose if weight and health goals have not yet been met.

Here's another way to think about it. All medications for any disease have "on-target" and "off-target" effects, meaning there are desirable benefits and some less-than-desirable ones. So, if you think about chemotherapy—we want the medicine to target the cancer cells (on-target effects), but in so doing, these medications can also cause nausea or vomiting (off-target effects). For obesity medications, some of the common on-target or desired effects include decreased appetite, decreased food noise, weight loss (in the weight reduction phase), and weight maintenance (in the weight plateau and maintenance phase); overall the on-target effect is to recalibrate and decrease the body fat set point. These are clearly benefits that we want to maximize. The undesirable effects, such as gastrointestinal side effects, if they arise, tend to go away once the swings in the concentration of the medicine in our body start to level off.

I am mentioning all of this because it can provide a strategy for avoiding or mitigating the undesirable side effects for those who experience them. As there is predictability in when side effects occur and how long they last, we have an opportunity to make things better by taking things more slowly. Right now we don't know who will and won't have side effects until they take the medicine. This is no different from medicine for any other disease.

The "Oops" Moments

Let's imagine going away for a two-week vacation, but you forgot your medicine (oops!). Or maybe it is not an "oops" moment but somewhat intentional, as it was for Todd, a thirty-eight-year-old math teacher with obesity and gout. A few days after he first started his medication, prescribed to him by his forward-thinking primary care provider, he went with friends to get hot wings, his favorite treat. He ate just a couple of wings slathered in spicy buffalo sauce and couldn't stomach one more. He was miserable all night. The thought of anything spicy made him want to vomit, and he swore he would not take another dose because the nausea was so bad. But a few days later, he was feeling much better, had already started losing weight, and thought that maybe he would give it another try. He had symptoms a few days after his second injection, but they were not nearly as bad. He also knew to opt for something more mild than the spicy wings the day or two around his injection. The day after his fourth injection of the lowest dose, he still had pretty notable nausea symptoms, so he and his provider decided to wait another month before increasing to the next dose.

Over the next several months, he worked with his doctor to increase the dose of medication. Slowly but surely, he lost thirty-four pounds. His nausea resolved. He was happy with his progress; even his gout seemed to get better with fewer flares. He felt great and was really pleased with his response to the medication.

Todd loved to travel south during his spring break, and well before he started the medication, he had booked a ten-day all-inclusive vacation at a resort on a Caribbean island. He could not wait to go on the trip. He had even invested in a fresh summer wardrobe to fit his new proportions. Then he remembered from years past that there would be twenty-four-foot-long buffet spreads and tiered dessert tables and tropical cocktails. Todd had already paid for the all-you-can-eat goodies, and, given the price tag, he wanted to maximize the value of his trip, even if it meant gaining back a few pounds.

Todd decided that he would not take his medication the night before he left and would not bring it with him. He would eat, drink, be merry, and get his money's worth at the same time. He planned to resume the medication after returning home.

When he arrived, he saw all the fabulous food everywhere, but somehow he was not interested in it. This reaction did not bother him; he just didn't care for it one way or another. This should not be much of a surprise, because the amount of medication in his body was still quite high. He snorkeled, played water volleyball, sat by the poolside and read, and even learned how to swing dance (the first time he'd ever been interested in signing up for the lessons). He had a fantastic time! The main difference was that his interest in the sweets and raw bar was muted. If he had dessert, one small slice of rum cake, or even just part of one, was definitely enough. Toward the end of his vacation (when the amount of medication in his body was half of what it was a week prior), some of the goodies started faintly calling his name, but he had a bite or two of caramelized plantains and then quickly moved on.

When Todd returned home, he was expecting the worst when he weighed himself. Finally, he got up the courage and stepped onto his scale. He was startled to find that his weight was exactly what it had been before he left for the island. He started to cry. He had not lost any more weight, but he certainly had not gained any weight.

Todd thought: "Maybe I'm cured? My doctor told me that I would always have to take these medications, but maybe I'm different." He was thrilled! And so, he decided to skip one more injection (three weeks total, so basically a month completely off his medication).

By the end of that month, Todd's medication levels were about 5% of what they had been a few weeks ago. His hunger came back with a fury because his body fat sct point was raised back up, the feedback loop signaling that he was starving and needed to store more fat, more fuel, more energy to reach his higher Enough Point (and to do that, his weight would need to get back to being thirty-four pounds heavier!). He started to eat more, and then eat everything in sight, including the hot wings. It didn't take long for him to start gaining back the weight, and the next time he stepped onto the scale he saw he had gained back about ten pounds.

Todd felt ashamed and was super self-critical. He had already taken the tags off the pricey designer clothing he had bought on his trip (as well as what he had purchased before). He also didn't want his friends, family, and doctor to blame him for messing up. All this reminded him that he had obesity, a chronic disease that must be treated chronically, and so he needed the medication to maintain his weight and health goals.

Unfortunately, this was not the end of the challenging part of Todd's experience. He was embarrassed by what had happened, and he had forgotten the part about reaching out to his doctor when things were going poorly. Instead, after much agonizing, he walked to the fridge, took out his medication, and gave himself a shot. Uh-oh . . . Now remember, he was on a relatively high dose of medication that had taken him several months to work up to in the setting of nausea.

Sometime after he took his injection, Todd initially started to feel better. The food noise diminished, and his cravings quieted. He was happy to feel full and satisfied after a small dinner, and he went to bed feeling relief that he was again treating his obesity. Early in the morning, he felt nauseated and woozy. He got up, ran into the bathroom to vomit, and continued to vomit every few hours. He called in sick for work, and over the next twenty-four hours, he couldn't keep much of anything down. When he got up from bed, he felt lightheaded. Todd called his sister to take him to urgent care, where they gave him intravenous fluids for dehydration and some nausea medicine. Eventually, he started feeling better and was able to drink some Gatorade and keep down a few saltines. Then he had to wait it out, until the levels of medicine started to come down again from the very high dose that he had taken.

So what just happened? Our brilliant bodies want to keep within certain ranges or norms, as that is where they feel and function best. So, our bodies do not like sudden changes; they like slow, sustained change and try to protect us against rapid disruptions. Todd restarting his relatively high dose of medication after missing several injections was a jolt to his system.

It took Todd days to get back to baseline. Even though the vomiting stopped and nausea subsided, he had little interest in food and was afraid to restart his medication for a while. Once his doctor explained to him what happened, he agreed to restart on the lowest dose again, and over several months he was able to go back up to the dose he had previously been taking.

He eventually required going up to the highest dose and stabilized his weight after losing about forty-four pounds. He did need to make some additional wardrobe purchases, including a new belt, but was very pleased with how he felt overall: His health had improved and his gout had all but resolved.

Less Common Side Effects

Quisha was very happy with her progress on the new medications for obesity treatment but thought perhaps she could do it "better and faster." She maintained her intense exercise program with a goal to help the pounds come off faster. A self-proclaimed type A professional in her late thirties, she had tried everything to lose weight and was amazed at how much easier it was for her to stick to her eating plan. She tolerated the medication well, with minimal side effects, although she did notice she was losing some hair. She lost nearly fifty pounds in six months. Her rate of a little more than two pounds per week was quite fast—she was losing more than 1% of her body weight per week.

Then Quisha started feeling a bit off. Initially, it felt like a slight pain in her belly that she couldn't identify, and it grew worse when she ate fatty foods. She pushed on while taking care to avoid fats. She felt tired, and her abdominal pain—in the middle of her torso and slightly to the right side—became more distinct. Eventually, she became worried when the pain intensified, and she went to the emergency room, where they performed an ultrasound of her abdomen. The radiologist saw that her gallbladder was inflamed, full of gallstones, and needed to come out. She was admitted to the hospital for laparoscopic removal of her gallbladder with all those little stones. The surgery went well, and she was feeling much better shortly thereafter.

Quisha was able to resume her medication, but this time, she was much more cautious. She worked with her provider to increase the dose back up slowly. Her rate of weight loss was now about half a pound per week. She was careful to stay well hydrated, avoided fatty foods for a while longer, and continued to exercise, but she changed the goal from burning as many calories as possible to having fun, feeling great, maintaining her muscle strength and flexibility, and improving her health. I include the side effect of gallstones because, although it is rare, it does happen.

Gallstones and inflammation of the gallbladder (cholecystitis) can occur with any form of rapid weight loss—bariatric surgery, caloric restriction, and effective medications. Now that these newer medications are achieving degrees of weight reduction that are similar to those achieved with bariatric surgery, we should not be surprised that we are seeing some similar side effects. The way these medications work may also directly impact gallbladder function, increasing the possibility of developing gallstones. Obesity in and of itself is also a risk factor for gallbladder disease, as is being female or over age forty. If gallstones occur, the presenting symptom is often abdominal pain, which can be accompanied by decreased food intake, at times vomiting, and sometimes fever. If gallstones are found in the setting of these symptoms, then the gallbladder needs to be surgically removed, usually by a laparoscopic procedure. Once the issue is resolved and the patient has recovered, it is generally considered safe to restart the medications—of course, under the health care provider's guidance.

If you do experience abdominal pain, tell your health care provider or go to an emergency room, where gallstones or other causes for the pain can be evaluated. Rarely, pancreatitis (an inflammation of the pancreas) is identified. While rare, this is more common in people with diabetes, who have an increased baseline risk of developing pancreatitis. High alcohol use, high triglyceride levels, and having gallstones can also increase the possibility of having pancreatitis. Rarely there are elevations in liver enzymes, but in general these medications help the liver by decreasing the amount of fat that is inappropriately stored there (the liver moonlights as a fat pantry).

Since the introduction of GLP-1-based medication (and DPP-4 inhibitors) for the treatment of diabetes, in addition to monitoring for pancreatitis, there has also been monitoring for cancer in the trials. Twenty years later there is no signal to suggest that cancer risk increases. Meaning that similar numbers of people who do and don't take these medications will get cancer, but overall there is no meaningful difference.

Special attention has been given to thyroid cancer, which is an obesity-related cancer. This means that having obesity increases your risk of getting thyroid cancer, specifically papillary thyroid cancer, which also happens to be the most common type of thyroid cancer. We don't know yet if treating obesity early and over a lifetime will decrease the risk of developing obesity-related cancers, including papillary thyroid cancers. To answer this important question, we will need to conduct very large trials and follow participants for years. Thyroid cancer has become a recurring question from patients in the setting of these medications because on the label there is a warning pertaining to medullary thyroid carcinoma, which is a rarer subtype of thyroid cancer, different from the more common papillary form. Why does this warning exist?

Years ago, animal studies found C-cell hyperplasia (an overgrowth of cells that eventually can lead to medullary thyroid cancer) and tumors in rats and mice who were given a GLP-1 receptor agonist. Rodents have a lot of GLP-1 receptors on their C-cells, whereas other animal species, including nonhuman primates (monkeys) and humans, do not. When the medicine was given to monkeys at very high doses (more than sixty times what would be given to a human) they did not develop C-cell hyperplasia or tumors. Because the finding was identified in two species, mice and rats, the medicines are contraindicated in people who have a higher baseline risk of medullary thyroid cancer (the type that relates to C cells), namely people with a family history of medullary thyroid cancer and of multiple endocrine neoplasia (a genetic disease that includes medullary thyroid cancer as one of its features). Your health care provider will review your medical record and ask you if you have a personal or family history of these diseases if these medications are being considered for treatment of obesity, diabetes, heart problems, or any other disease.

Feeling Energized or Tired?

Although many patients may feel energized when they take these medications, fatigue (feeling tired) has been observed in some participants in the trials. We also see both improved energy levels as well as fatigue in our patients in the clinical setting. If a patient is experiencing fatigue, this may be due to eating much less or drinking less, especially during the initial few months of the weight reduction phase. Making sure to drink enough water can help prevent fatigue (and nausea, actually). It is also very important for your kidneys because it can protect them from injury that can occur if patients become dehydrated while taking these medications. If your appetite goes down a significant amount, it becomes that much more important to prioritize plenty of water and nutritious foods—lean protein, vegetables and fruits, and healthy fats—so that you don't miss out on vitamins and nutrients. If you have a really hard time eating much of anything, speak with your health care provider, because possibly you need a decrease in the dose of medication. The decrease in dose will likely be temporary and will not affect the ultimate amount of weight you lose, but what it will do is keep you healthy while you are losing weight. If you are eating very little, let your provider know so that they are aware and can help you.

There are other causes of fatigue. You may be eating and drinking an adequate amount, but for some, fatigue may be related to the medicine itself. The description of fatigue from patients varies: Sometimes it is described as decreased energy, brain fog, or just feeling like they have less "get up and go." If this occurs, let your provider know. They may lower the dose or, if the side effect does not subside, a medication change may be needed.

How's Your Mood?

As discussed in chapter 7, addressing mental health throughout obesity care is key. There are many psychosocial and psychological aspects of losing weight, and given the past history of medication for obesity treatment, mood has been something that has been monitored closely in clinical trials. Recent evaluations of available data by the European Medicines Agency (EMA) demonstrated no increase in thoughts of self-harm, and additional analyses found that NuSH-based medications are associated with improvement in mental-health-related quality of life. Additional research is needed in populations who have a psychiatric diagnosis at baseline. Bottom line, if you notice any mood changes, up or down, letting your provider know is very important. They are there to support you in getting the care you need.

What About Hair Loss?

Remember Quisha's hair loss in the setting of her weight reduction? This side effect is called telogen effluvium and is also seen in patients who have undergone bariatric surgery and experienced rapid weight loss. It occurs when stress, illness, or big life changes push more hairs than usual to shed at once—causing diffuse thinning that usually grows back over time. Childbirth, major surgery, significant psychological stress, or thyroid problems are all examples of things that can cause telogen effluvium. Hair growth usually resumes after weight has plateaued. If you're still losing hair several months after having stabilized your weight (and are eating and sleeping well), seeing a dermatologist may also be helpful to identify additional contributors and potential treatments.

Skin Reactions?

Some patients also may notice mild to moderate skin reactions (such as redness, itchiness) at the site of injections, which can be related to what the medication is dissolved in. This usually resolves on its own over time. If these do not go away over time and are severe enough, a different injectable medication or a change to an oral medication may be required, though this is rare.

More to Learn: Nutrition, Bones, Muscles, and More

Even though GLP-1 receptor agonists have been used for the treatment of type 2 diabetes for over twenty years, there is still much to be learned about these medications. The amount of weight lost with the newer-generation medications or with combination therapy is approaching that observed with bariatric surgery. Therefore it is important to consider that some of the adverse effects seen with bariatric surgery may emerge with medical treatment. These may include nutritional deficiencies (including vitamin deficiencies), decrease in bone density (bone loss) especially in older individuals, and changes in muscle mass, as discussed earlier. It is important to consider the potential benefits versus the potential risks when choosing treatments.

Risks Versus Benefits

As mentioned in earlier chapters, similar to any medical intervention, the treatment of obesity is about balancing risks versus benefits for each individual. These medications are not recommended for people who do not have obesity, or are overweight without other obesity-related diseases. Indications, such as type 2 diabetes, obstructive sleep apnea, as well as prevention of a second heart attack and stroke, will likely continue to accrue. Whether you have any of these obesity-related complications already or have obesity alone, your health care provider is continuously and carefully assessing (and reassessing) the risk versus benefit of any and all potential treatments.

When considering the risks of treating obesity, remember there are also dangers in not addressing it. In addition to a shortened life expectancy for those with severe obesity, if obesity is left untreated, its consequences and impact on daily life can increase. This includes nonmedical concerns—everything from tying your shoes to carrying groceries up the stairs, feeling breathless with minimal activity, or experiencing joint or back pain. There's also the food noise, the cognitive load, and the mental and emotional weight of shame and blame.

Our bodies compensate for as long as they can, but obesity-related complications like heart disease, kidney disease, and certain types of cancer can emerge. We also see this in adolescents and children with severe obesity who develop type 2 diabetes, high blood pressure, and kidney disease at an early age. The prevalence of childhood type 2 diabetes continues to increase, paralleling the increase in rates of obesity and underscoring the need for effective early interventions, including with obesity medications.

The goal of evaluating the side effects of the medication *and* the risks of obesity is to give our patients a complete picture, which is crucial for making well-informed decisions. As we've discussed, most people do not experience significant side effects, and there are many ways to work through them if they do occur. Rarely, there are patients whose side effects persist even at the lowest doses, and in those cases, we try switching therapies, or further slowing down when increasing the dose.

Given that side effects vary dramatically from patient to patient, I invite my patients to share their experiences with me so that we can work through them together from the beginning. The invitation to share side effects is important because sometimes the motivation to lose weight is so great that a person may want to endure side effects and not share them for fear that the medication will be stopped. I reassure my patients that whatever is going on, we'll figure it out together, and we'll find the treatment path that meets their needs and goals.

That was the case with my patient Carla, who mentions she is worried about side effects. One of her friends had significant nausea when she started taking one of the medications, but when I ask about dosage, Carla shares that she was not sure if her friend started with the lowest dose. Carla and I talk about the different ways we can help prevent and ease side effects if she chooses to pursue treatment. She feels reassured and is comfortable asking more questions, which we discuss and address one by one.

10

You Are Enough

Hope, Health, and the Future of Obesity Treatment

In January 2025, I was asked to speak at an event that was a little different from my usual presentations: It was not for a gathering of international scientists and clinicians but for a general audience, and it was not going to be held at a convention center but at Lincoln Center in New York City. I was excited to be able to share the story of my patients' biology with a wider audience. I knew that I wanted to inspire the attendees of the Yale For Humanity event to pause and consider that obesity is and always has been a disease, and that if we treat this one disease effectively, we can change the face of medicine. That was my goal. I wanted to stand on that stage and share that together we can transform the health of our patients, health care, and someday, the health of the world.

But how to do that? With her permission, I had shared Alice's story of losing over ninety pounds many times before. But this talk was for a general audience, not medical or scientific colleagues. I wondered if I should add photos to convey Alice's journey, not just BMI line graphs of her weight and treatment trajectory over time. After all, photos introduce another level of storytelling . . . and, perhaps more important, human vulnerability. I asked Alice what she thought about sharing her image, letting her know that this talk would be recorded and posted online . . . available to the world. What did she think of the idea of sharing her photos, and would she be comfortable with such exposure?

She instantly agreed. She has been very open about having obesity, her struggles with it, and how she had come to Y-Weight, in her words, "desperately" seeking help. Being a part of this trial and finding an effective medication had transformed her life. Her desire to help others by sharing her years of battling her weight, the experience of participating in the trial, and the challenges when the study ended overpowered any concern that her body (and face) would be out there for the world to see. Our goals were aligned. We both wanted to impact meaningful change in how obesity is perceived and how treatment options are understood. This talk and her images would be a powerful way to not just inform people's minds but impact their hearts as well.

I chose several photos to depict her journey and completed the slide with two more—one of Alice at the start of the trial, and one at its end. I included her BMI-over-time graph and sent the slide for her review. She called me to approve it and, in the same breath, said, "You know, it's not about the before-and-after selfie."

She was absolutely right.

It is *not* about the before and after.

It is about the process. It is about health—mental and physical. It's about self-compassion and self-love. Alice knew and had internalized that her treatment was not about crossing an imaginary finish line. Gaining and keeping health is not about two snapshots, two moments in time. It's about a whole life, an ongoing pursuit . . . yes, a journey.

When I see any before-and-after photos of patients who lost weight with these new obesity medicines, I think about all that came in between those two snapshots. I think about what the person may have felt, experienced, endured, and overcome. I also think of all that is to come—the next "after" and each of the "afters" that follow.

What's Next? A Glimpse Into the Future

Obesity treatment is rapidly transforming before our eyes. This book is a snapshot of a moment in time in 2025 in the midst of this remarkable revolution. I asked a few of my senior medical colleagues to share with me what they are excited about for the future of our patients, for the treatment of obesity, especially given their perspective over many decades, so you'll see some of their comments in this chapter as well.

In this book we've discussed the current NuSH-based medications and researchers around the world are working on developing countless more that target different hormone pathways. For instance, at Y-Weight, we are currently studying a triple receptor agonist, retatrutide, which looks to be approaching the amount of weight reduction that is seen with bariatric surgery. It targets three hormone receptors for three different hormones: GIP, GLP-1, and glucagon. For an earlier development phase 2 study of retatrutide, I presented the results at the ADA Scientific Sessions meeting in June 2023.

Admittedly, when I first saw the results months prior, I nearly fell out of my chair, especially seeing those for women who had higher BMI (≥35 kg/m²) at baseline: This subgroup lost approximately 30% of their body weight on treatment with retatrutide. I will always remember the moment I shared the full cohort's efficacy results: participants lost on average nearly 25% of their body weight (on average fifty-eight pounds) in eleven months. The audience clapped *in the middle of the presentation*! I don't think I've ever seen that happen before, certainly not in the middle of one of my presentations. But that day the normally sober-minded, eminently logical, and usually unflappable researchers and clinicians in that auditorium *clapped*, because these results were just that impressive. The phase 3 trials with this triple hormone agonist are ongoing, and once the trials have completed, the FDA will soon have the safety and efficacy data it needs to review this new agent as a potential therapeutic option for the treatment of obesity.

What is very key are the broader health benefits that come with obesity treatment with different agents. In the case of retatrutide, the targeting of the glucagon receptor may offer an added advantage: supporting liver health, on top of the other improvements we're already seeing. There are also dual receptor agonists being developed—such as survodutide, pemvidutide, and mazdutide, which target the glucagon receptor (and the GLP-1 receptor) and thus may also benefit the liver. And with other agents in development, there are innumerable potential health benefits yet to be explored.

There are many new innovations in the pipeline: For example, at Y-Weight, we're studying other novel combinations of NuSH receptor modulators such as CagriSema, which activates both GLP-1 and amylin receptors, and survodutide, which activates both GLP-1 and glucagon receptors. Given that these medications are branching out to target other combinations of NuSH receptors, they may enable new health benefits, expand the amount of weight loss, and differ in tolerability and efficacy for various types of obesity. We're also studying MariTide, which is a potential monthly injectable medication that combines GLP-1 receptor agonism with GIP receptor antagonism. Imagine taking twelve shots a year, just one per month or maybe even fewer, to effectively treat obesity. With some agents we are also conducting trials in younger patients—adolescents and children who have severe obesity. Leaving obesity untreated in younger patients can predispose them to developing "adult" diseases even while they are still children, necessitating a lifetime of intensive medical treatments.

The next wave of treatment innovation to come is the ability to deliver these medications as pills or capsules, rather than as injections: Oral semaglutide and orforglipron are two medicines that are the farthest along. Oral semaglutide has been FDA approved for the treatment of diabetes for several years, and now a higher dose is under review by the FDA for the treatment of obesity. Orforglipron, the first small-molecule GLP-1-based medication, demonstrated promising results both in terms of weight and hemoglobin A1c reduction and is under review by the FDA for obesity treatment, as well as for diabetes. Because orforglipron is a small molecule, rather than a peptide, it can be taken without food or water restrictions (it is not chewed up by our digestive enzymes).

"The availability of new oral medications that are effective, safe, easier to distribute, and (hopefully) lower in cost will change the treatment paradigm," says Dr. Lou Aronne, ". . . so that people can be treated earlier, before developing the many complications of obesity. In addition, people without access will be able to be treated." Currently, about a quarter of the world's population has obesity, so there is a great need for accessible treatment options. Oral medications, specifically small molecules, are often simpler and potentially less expensive to manufacture than the injectable peptides, their supply is more easily scalable, they are easier to transport and store with no refrigeration needed, thus providing us with the opportunity to treat obesity around the world.

Moreover, there are clues from our clinical patients that may help us consider additional uses for NuSH-based obesity medications and investigate the biological processes that may impact other medical conditions. Early studies suggest they may help people with alcohol-use disorder want to drink less alcohol. In conjunction with other medications, they may help allay dementia or inflammatory conditions like psoriatic arthritis. We need to continue to do the research to better understand how these medications impact the biology of these other diseases.

Given the complexity of obesity and the variability in response—some people lose a substantial amount of weight, while others lose hardly any weight—we need a wider range of options. In other words, more tools in our toolbox to better individualize care. For a look at the next potential wave of NuSH-based obesity medications that are being developed and are already pretty far along (phase 3), check out the table in the Appendix on page 244. There are also hundreds of medications in earlier development (phase 2, phase 1, and preclinical). Some target NuSH pathways, while others target completely different biological mechanisms, forming distinctly new classes of medications for the treatment of obesity.

One such new class of medications being explored are medications which could help preserve muscle mass. People with obesity in general have more muscle mass as they need to carry more weight against gravity. With any form of weight loss (diet, medications, surgery), both fat and lean mass, including muscle, are lost. A goal would be to lose predominantly fat, as that's what's causing the negative downstream health effects, and preserve the lean mass, including muscle and bone. One category of new medications includes myostatin-activin pathway inhibitors (MAPi). Although these medications do not result in as much overall weight reduction (in part because building muscle increases lean mass), they do result in significant fat loss. When used in combination with a NuSH-based medication, they may be able to limit weight reduction to mainly loss of fat while preserving muscle. This has been shown with the weekly injectable agent bimagrumab, which is the farthest along in development in this potential new class of medications. Wouldn't that be good—to lose mostly fat but not muscle?

Innumerable additional new classes of medications and treatment strategies are rapidly evolving, targeting distinctly different biological mechanisms, bringing with them hope and promise for effective treatment options for our patients. These are treatments that target the biology of obesity and improve overall health. Dr. Donna Ryan summed it up best. "Let's get real," she said. "I never dreamed that our work to identify medications to help patients lose weight would result in a class of drugs that goes beyond weight loss to reduce heart attack, stroke, need for dialysis and CPAP, heart failure symptoms and hospitalizations, COVID deaths, and *more*. It's not a dream come true—it's beyond my wildest imaginings." Dr. Harlan Krumholz added, "For the first time, we are seeing treatments for obesity that don't just help people lose weight—they help them gain health. This is a turning point in medicine and in how society understands obesity."

Dr. Lee Kaplan added, "With the tremendous ability of these drugs to improve or control so many of the complications of obesity, it is only a matter of time until we learn which cancers can be effectively prevented by them." He paused and added, "We don't yet understand exactly how these medications work so effectively to control obesity, but they will eventually reveal their secret. And when they do, they will give us important clues as to how to prevent obesity in the first place, which will be an even greater benefit to society."

Imagine that. Imagine a world where we can prevent obesity.

Ted Kyle, of ConscienHealth, summarized: "The reason all of this scientific progress is so exciting is that it has started a shift in the culture toward understanding obesity for what it is: a biological problem, not a behavioral or personal failure. This is hugely important."

These transformative, highly effective medications will enable the safe and effective treatment of obesity for mothers, fathers, sons, and daughters, aunts, nephews, friends, and neighbors. Hopefully they will allow them to experience a most common sentiment that my patients share with me—freedom.

To feel free! Overwhelmingly free. It's the most extraordinary experience to observe—it usually happens with my patients as they are losing weight, before they settle into their weight plateau. When all this is new, and they experience the world in a new light, just free.

The "so free" comes out in many ways, big and little.

- "Wrapping a bath towel around my whole body feels fantastic!"
- "Tying my shoes. I can tie my shoes."
- "I enjoy food without emotional turmoil; without feeling guilty for eating one cheesy nacho. I can go out with my friends and just enjoy our time together."
- "Crossing my legs. Now I'm part of the club."
- "Walking into any clothing store and finding things in my size. Like everywhere. At first it was weird and now it feels normal."
- "I stopped having to take [multiple daily] insulin shots, and somehow my blood sugars are in normal range."
- "I can actually finally hear my thoughts now that the food noise is gone."

With treatment that targeted her biology, as Oprah said, she found her own freedom, and this newfound freedom had unexpected ripples ...

Oprah: I've found you just have so much more energy to offer yourself, and so much more energy to offer other people. All that energy I spent on "What am I gonna eat? What am I not gonna eat? What am I gonna eat next? What did I just eat? What shouldn't I have eaten?" has somehow been channeled into a desire to experience life differently. It has made me more spontaneous, more open to things I wouldn't have otherwise tried. I recently went to a bluegrass festival by myself. I woke up in Colorado one day and thought, "I'd like to do that." So I did. In this later part of my life, as I mentioned, it's opened up the aperture of adventure and possibility and new experiences. It's remarkable. I have long believed that the greatest aspiration that anyone can hold in this lifetime is to become more of yourself. Not to become more of what other people want, or what other people desire. The greatest aspiration is "How do you become more of yourself?"

What I know is that we're all striving for the same thing. And what do we want? We want to be able to live out the truest, purest, highest possibility of ourselves as human beings. And what this medicine allows me to do is to reach another level of that possibility, without having to strive for it, battle for it, fight my own self for it. It's just there, because all the crap, the angst, the cloudiness, the fuzziness, the worry that I've spent on my weight–that's energy. Anxiously anticipating what the next meal was going to be or what it was going to do to me, or how it was going to affect my body, and the guilt and the shame and all of that–that's energy too. Now that I've released it, I am free–to behold whatever is new and possible for myself. That is what happens with this medicine. It opens the aperture of hope and possibility. To literally hold the space for something new to come in.

Final Thoughts

That freedom. That hope. The possibility and space for something new to come in. I see this in my patients. You've now seen it too, in the stories that Oprah has shared, and the stories that Alice, Lynn, and so many others have shared.

The struggles and triumphs of people living with obesity can teach us, as my patients have taught me, how, together, we might shift the narrative about this disease. Shift away from shame and blame to compassionate care; understanding that obesity is a disease and not something anyone chooses. We can offer empathy to anyone who has been fighting their own brain and body and Enough Point. We now have the tools to help people with obesity recalibrate their Enough Point and treat the disease.

Some may choose to pursue treatment, and some may not—this is up to the person and what is right for their life.

There is certainly no one right answer for everybody. There is the right answer for you and your life, your health, and this may change and shift over your lifetime.

What is needed for everyone, every person at every size and every shape, is compassionate care.

Let's touch base one final time with Carla at the end of her first visit with me. She has wiped her eyes again, tucked in her blouse, and recomposed herself. There is a new sparkle of hope in her eyes. The anxiety of being late for a meeting at her office seems less important. After a long discussion together, she's decided to try a weekly medication. She'll begin at the lowest starting dose and will communicate with me if she experiences issues. She is aware of the potentially more serious but rare side effects to look out for as well as the more common ones and strategies to manage them with my help. She has rummaged through her cupboard at home to search for her pale purple Yeti tumbler to fill with water and drink from daily. She will prioritize protein and fiber and think about the nutrition and energy she will get from them. She starts to walk toward checkout to arrange for the first of many follow-up appointments to come. She turns and says, "Thank you, Dr. Ania!" I smile at her, pause for a moment, then head in to see my next patient who is here for a return follow-up visit. I look at her vitals in the chart before I knock on the door.

Even though it is just a number, it is a measure and gives me a hint that she's starting to respond to her treatment. I am so privileged to share in all my patients' lives and so grateful that they entrust me with their care.

Now let's fast-forward in time with Carla to where she is now, two years later: She has lost and maintained seventy pounds of her eighty-pound goal. She had not recognized it before the medication, but she had been experiencing very significant food noise that vanished after her first few doses. She reports that her productivity has increased. She still does not enjoy driving on I-95, but now sings on the way up to her visits. She knows the highway as a predictable obstacle, but she also feels braced to manage it and the many other challenges, emotions, and adventures that await her. She knows there are more tools in the obesity treatment toolbox, and we'll keep going—who knows, there may even be another wardrobe change. But for now she is satisfied, her hip pain has resolved, and her back pain has improved as she continues physical therapy sessions. With fewer aches, she started salsa classes with her husband. They are taking their three young adult sons for a once-in-a-lifetime hiking trip to Peru. Carla's life isn't perfect. Her job is still stressful (though she loves it), her hair has thinned with the weight loss and menopause, and her youngest son still "forgets" to clean his room. But Carla has made the shift away from shame and blame, away from frustration and hopelessness. She understands she has a disease—a treatable disease—and it's the disease of obesity.

From Carla's story and Oprah's story and the many patient stories in this book, I hope you take away this: Obesity is a chronic disease, not a choice. Treating obesity is a lifelong process. If you choose to have treatment there are safe and effective options. We now know that targeting the biology to recalibrate the Enough Point treats the disease itself—and that this can also prevent and treat hundreds of other obesity-related conditions. With continued research and compassionate care for all people living with obesity, we have the potential to change the health of our world . . . by treating one disease, one *person* at a time.

Now that really would be . . . *enough.*

Acknowledgments

With deep gratitude, to all the participants in all the trials, to all the patients who entrust us with their care and their health, this book would not have been possible without you. By vulnerably sharing your stories, you have taught us to listen, to hear, to hold compassion for your silent pain.

To Oprah Winfrey, for turning your own pain and public shaming into an empathetic gift for all those living with obesity. Your idea for this book turned into reality. Without you, this book would not exist.

To Tara Montgomery, Nicole Nichols, Brian Piotrowicz, Brad Pavone, Erinn McNeill, and Chelsea Hettrick—you shaped the conversations that led to this book.

To Bob Miller, for being the mastermind who brought all of us together, for your vision, and for always being relentlessly supportive.

To everyone at Avid Reader Press/Simon & Schuster: Jofie Ferrari-Adler, Ben Loehnen, Caroline Sutton, Megan Noes, Meredith Vilarello, Ilana Gold, Emily Lewis, Alison Forner, Clay Smith, Jessica Chin, Allison Green, and Ruth Lee-Mui.

To Cheryl Cronin, for coming over at the drop of a hat to take a beautiful (last-minute!) headshot in my backyard. To Henry, for bringing simplicity and beauty to the Enough Point figure.

For all the editorial support for a physician-scientist who knew only scientific writing. Leigh Newman, for your creativity and whimsicality; Leslie Wells, for your focus and attention to detail; Mamie Healey, for your eternally positive and attentive approach—you helped me bring this home. Dick Kibbey, you are not an editor but you made it your side gig above your own—I am grateful.

To my readers, you are incredible. Lee Kaplan, Lou Aronne, Donna Ryan, Glenda Callender, Elizabeth Rathbun, David Berg, Harlan Krumholz, Michelle Van Name, Ted Kyle, Joe Nadglowski, Lena Smith Parker, Chrissie: You are my village! Your insightful perspective and timely feedback helped evolve the manuscript with lightning speed.

To my mentors, sponsors, and colleagues RS and RS, LK, LA, DR, HK, NA, MC, and so many more, all of you gave me the freedom to do what I believed in and the support to know it was the right thing to do.

Mom and Dad and big bro, you gave me my "why" in life, my purpose; you laid the foundation through prioritizing education, work ethic, relationships, and meaning. I love you.

To Dick, my one-in-eight-billion, thoughtful, intelligent, perfect-for-me best friend, for always being there, always supporting me, always intuitively knowing just what I need. You are the reason I can do what I do. I'm the lucky one. I love you.

Author's Note

Dr. Jastreboff conducts multicenter trials with Amgen, Boehringer Ingelheim, Eli Lilly, Novo Nordisk, and Rhythm Pharmaceuticals; serves on scientific advisory boards for Amgen, AstraZeneca, Boehringer Ingelheim, Biohaven, Eli Lilly, IntelliHealth/Flyte, Metsera, Novo Nordisk, Pfizer, Regeneron, Roche, Scholar Rock, Structure Therapeutics, Syntis Bio, WW International, and Zealand Pharma; and is an academic cofounder of State 4 Therapeutics.

Appendix

Anticipated Potential New NuSH-Based Medications

These medications are far along in the process—phase 3 or FDA review—as of summer 2025.
They are anticipated to be potential new therapies in the next five to seven years.

NuSH-based medications for obesity in phase 3 or under FDA review				
Molecule name	Target	Mode of delivery	Frequency	Status
CagriSema	Amylin / calcitonin receptor agonist (cagrilintide)/ GLP-1 receptor agonist (semaglutide)	Injection	Weekly	FDA review 2026
Orforglipron	GLP-1 receptor agonist (small molecule)	Oral	Daily	FDA review 2025–2026
Semaglutide	GLP-1 receptor agonist (peptide)	Oral	Daily	FDA review 2025–2026
Retatrutide	Glucagon / GIP / GLP-1 receptor agonist	Injection	Weekly	Phase 3 trials ending 2025–2026
Survodutide	Glucagon / GLP-1 receptor agonist	Injection	Weekly	Phase 3 trials ending 2025–2026
MariTide	GIP receptor antagonist / GLP-1 receptor agonist (maridebart cafraglutide)	Injection	Monthly	Phase 3 trials started in 2025
VK2735	GIP / GLP-1 receptor agonist	Injection	Weekly	Phase 3 trials started in 2025
CT-388	GIP / GLP-1 receptor agonist	Injection	Weekly	Phase 3 trials starting in 2026

MET-O97i	GLP-1 receptor agonist	Injection	Monthly	Phase 3 trials starting in 2026
Amycretin	Amylin / calcitonin and GLP-1 receptor agonist	Injection/oral	Weekly/daily	Phase 3 trials starting in 2026
Eloralintide	Amylin receptor agonist	Injection	Weekly	Phase 3 trials starting in 2026
Petrelintide	Amylin / calcitonin receptor agonist	Injection	Weekly	Phase 3 trials starting in 2026

*NuSH—nutrient-stimulated hormone

Hundreds of other agents are currently in earlier stages of development. These include both NuSH-based medications as well as medications that target completely new mechanisms. Stay tuned!

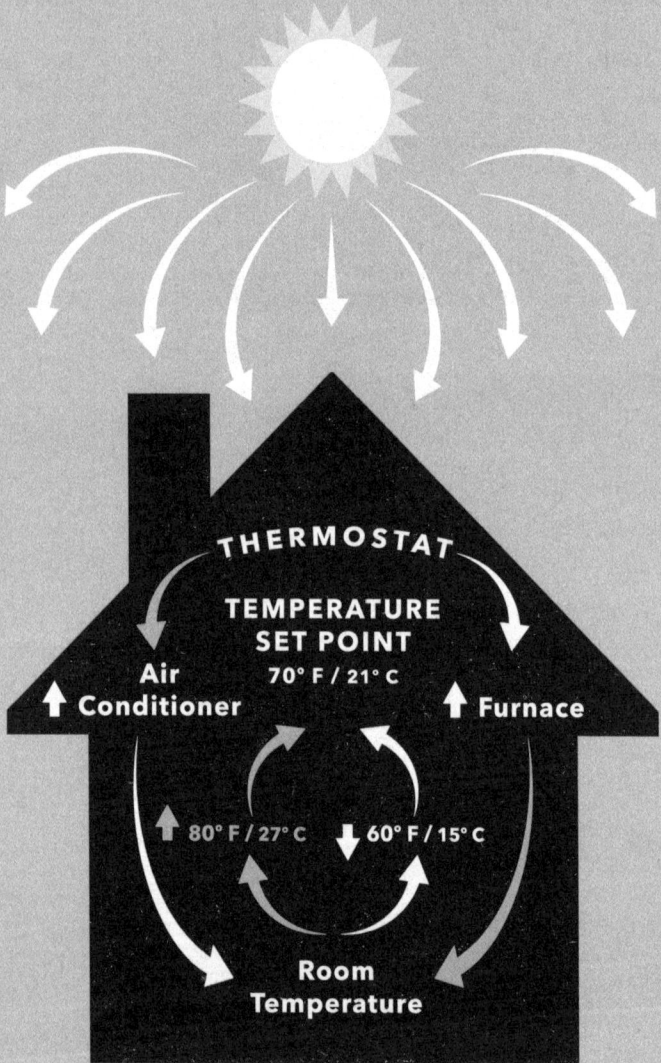

TEMPERATURE SET POINT

THERMOSTAT

TEMPERATURE
SET POINT
70° F / 21° C

Air
Conditioner

Furnace

80° F / 27° C   60° F / 15° C

Room
Temperature

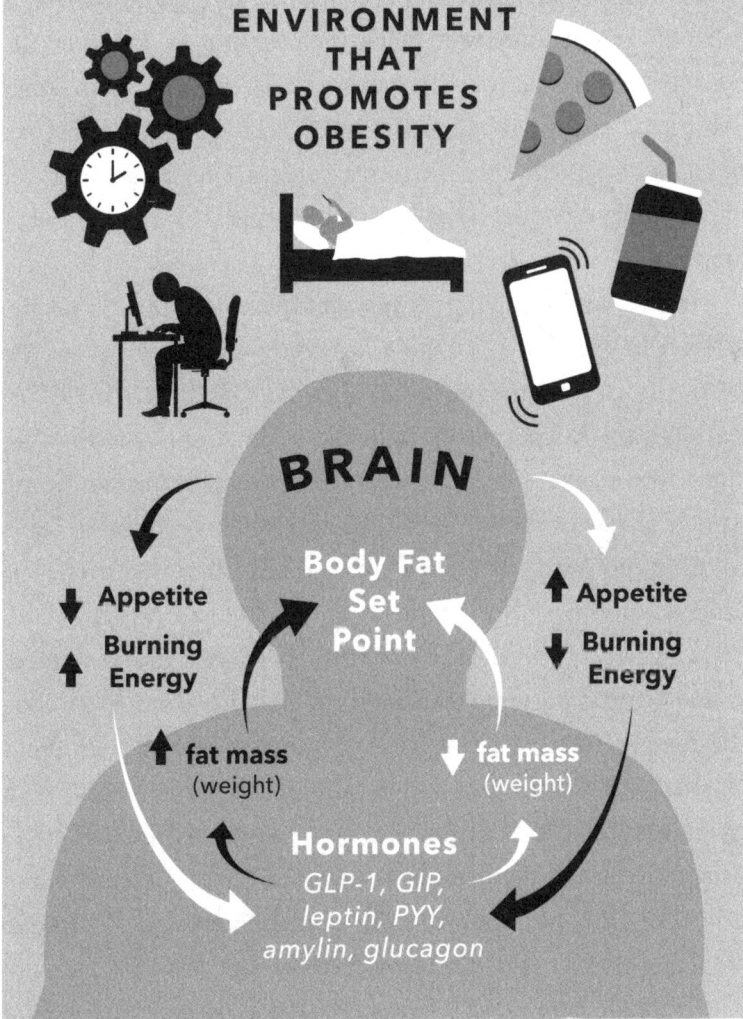

BODY FAT SET POINT
ENOUGH POINT

ENVIRONMENT THAT PROMOTES OBESITY

BRAIN

Body Fat Set Point

↓ Appetite
↑ Burning Energy

↑ Appetite
↓ Burning Energy

↑ fat mass (weight)

↓ fat mass (weight)

Hormones
GLP-1, GIP, leptin, PYY, amylin, glucagon

Figure Legend

The thermostat in the house senses the room temperature. If the sun is shining and raises the temperature across the entire house higher (warmer) than the thermostat setting of 70°F, then it triggers the AC to cool the room. Once the temperature is brought back to the temperature set point, the AC turns off. Likewise, if the room temperature were below the temperature set point, the thermostat would activate the furnace to warm the room. In either case, if the room temperature is at or near the temperature set point, neither the AC nor the furnace are on. Keeping the room at its set point can be achieved by either heating or cooling feedback loops.

In the case of the poorly placed kitchen thermostat (as described in chapter 3), if there are confusing signals (e.g., the oven, the candle, the sunlight, and the closed kitchen door) warming the kitchen more than the other rooms, the thermostat will cool the warmed kitchen to its temperature set point, while the rest of the house will be cooler. This mismatch leads to an inappropriately cooled living room when the kitchen is at its set point.

The body has regulatory systems to control the amount of stored fat that are similar to those we just discussed controlling the temperature in the house. Let's say the body fat set point (Enough Point) is set to a body weight of about 155 pounds for a given individual. It's Thanksgiving, and she eats a little more than usual, so her body secretes hormones like GLP-1, GIP, amylin, and others that tell her brain that she's had enough and it's time to stop. She doesn't get the second helping, but has some dessert. The extra food energy (calories) get stored as extra fat, and her fat stores go up to 158 pounds by the end of the holiday. The extra fat secretes extra leptin, which travels through the blood to tell her brain (Enough Point) that she is storing too much energy. The response is a decrease in appetite and an increase in energy burning (metabolism), and so over the next few days her weight settles back down to its Enough Point at 155 pounds. The return to the Enough Point would also occur if her weight dropped (she was so busy with work, she did not have time to eat much for several days). In response to the loss of weight (specifically fat) her hunger would increase and her energy expenditure would decrease bringing her weight back up to her Enough Point.

Now, let's say the environment (filled with ultra-processed food, lack of physical activity and sleep, and lots of stress) has, over decades, pushed up her Enough Point to 211 pounds. As long as her actual weight was 211 pounds, then she would not feel hungry or stuffed and her energy expenditure would be normal for her. Now, she does not want her weight to be 211, so she consciously limits her food intake and increases her physical activity and loses 10 pounds. Her Enough Point says, "Hey, I am supposed to be at 211, so I am going to slow down your metabolism and increase your hunger, cravings, and food noise to try to bring your weight back to 211 pounds." Over time her weight would inch back up. Imagine if she had lost twenty or thirty pounds or more; the symptoms would be even greater the further she is below her Enough Point. The more weight she loses, the harder the Enough Point works to bring her body up to where the brain thinks it should be. Fortunately, instead of trying to fight the brain when her weight is 191 pounds (twenty pounds below her Enough Point), she takes one of the obesity medications that actually lowers her Enough

Point to 170 pounds. Because now her body is reporting to her brain that she is now twenty-one pounds over where she should be, it decreases her appetite and increases her energy expenditure until her body gets down to her Enough Point. At her Enough Point, she returns to a regular appetite and metabolism as long as she stays on the medication.

Additional Resources

Here is additional information about ongoing obesity research as well as national and international societies and associations that have resources about obesity. This list includes various societies and associations which focus fully or in part on obesity—hosting scientific meetings and educational courses, developing guidelines and standards of care, and advocating for people living with obesity.

To search for the latest obesity clinical trials: ClinicalTrials.gov

For additional information about the Yale Obesity Research Center (Y-Weight): https://medicine.yale.edu/yweight

Obesity
  The Obesity Society
  European Association for the Study of Obesity
  Obesity Canada
  World Obesity Federation
  Obesity Action Coalition
  Obesity Medicine Association
  American Board of Obesity Medicine

Centers for Disease Control and Prevention (CDC) obesity
website

National Institutes of Health/National Institute of Diabetes
and Digestive and Kidney Diseases (NIH/NIDDK) website
and workshops

World Health Organization (WHO)

Pediatric Endocrinology, General Pediatrics, and Obesity

American Academy of Pediatrics

Pediatric Endocrine Society

Type 2 Diabetes, Type 1 Diabetes, and Obesity

American Diabetes Association

European Association for the Study of Diabetes

Endocrine Disorders, Diabetes, and Obesity

Endocrine Society

American Association of Clinical Endocrinology

Heart Disease and Obesity

American Heart Association

American College of Cardiology

European Society of Cardiology

Cancer

American Cancer Society

American Association for Cancer Research

Women's Health

American College of Obstetricians and Gynecologists

Many more societies are rapidly developing an interest in obesity, so please stay tuned!

Notes

Chapter 2

39 *or the sex, age*

In children and adolescents, age and sex is accounted for in BMI percentiles.

45 *hungry all the time*

Monogenic forms of obesity, such as leptin deficiency, cause hyperphagia, which is an intense, persistent sensation of hunger that is insatiable.

52 *Fat can store more energy than sugar*

We all still need to have some energy in reserve—and we put it in fat cells. Although fat cells do many things (produce hormones like leptin, serve as thermal insulation for the body, protect organs, even play a role in immune function), the main purpose of fat cells is the essential role of storing fat. In fact, each adipocyte (fat cell) is filled with a giant lipid droplet that occupies about 90–95% of the cell volume, with a few mitochondria and a nucleus crammed in the remaining space. The lipid droplet has all the water-loving glycerol parts of the triglyceride on the rim of the sphere, while the greasy water-hating part is scrunched up tightly and buried in the core of the droplet. As opposed to glycogen, by keeping the water *out* of the blob, lipid droplets keep the lipids nice and compact (the opposite of our earlier overcooked pasta). Thousands of individual adipocytes congregate together to form what is known as a lobule of white adipose tissue (it's white because of the paucity of mitochondria, which otherwise would impart a reddish hue). As an example, think of a dry-aged, marbled rib-eye steak—it is easy to distinguish between the fat and the meat, based on the difference in color.

52 *4 kilocalories of energy*

Kilocalories are a unit of energy and—fun fact—kilocalories are represented as plain old calories on food labels.

53 *we would die*

Let's think about what happens to our energy balance throughout the day. As mentioned, glucose is an essential source of energy. It is in our bloodstream, which means that it can travel all over the body. We can get it to where we need it—our muscles, our brain, our organs—and we can get it there fast. Whether you spend your morning shopping, fishing, or going back to sleep, as your body digests that buttery bacon-egg-and-cheese breakfast croissant, you can count on glucose to be available to fuel these activities. When we're awake and eating every few hours, our body has readily available energy from the nutrients we just ingested. Remember, we have about a couple of wild-cherry Life Savers' worth of sugar in our blood at any one time. If we consume more energy than we need for that moment, then our body stores it for later use.

We do not have batteries, solar panels, hydroelectric dams, or nuclear reactors in our bodies to provide energy, so we have to rely on the energy generated from the burning (oxidation) of macronutrients. Essentially, our bodies are combustion engines: We consume food as fuel, breathe in oxygen, and exhale carbon dioxide and water as byproducts. That is why we breathe fast when we exercise; we need to take in more oxygen to burn macronutrients, and at the same time blow off the carbon dioxide waste that is produced. When it's time to generate energy, it's mitochondria that do the hard work. Mitochondria are everywhere in our body. Sugar and fat obtained from our food power our mitochondrial ATP nanofactories. Those little wormy things famous for being the "powerhouse of the cell" utilize a series of electrical and chemical reactions to extract the energy from metabolizing the fat and sugar in order to synthesize adenosine triphosphate—which we call ATP.

Think of ATP as similar to a power outlet in the wall that supports all sorts of important appliances: a charger that can make ice cubes in the freezer or, alternatively, warm a frozen burrito bowl with microwaves or power a reading lamp while you curl up with this book. With the correct adapter, it can charge your phone or electric toothbrush. ATP is the chemical currency that our cells use to perform a multitude of activities of daily living: writing poems, hanging streamers, laughing while simultaneously sighing at dad jokes, and smelling the rain. ATP is our body's chemical energy, the common fuel that we make from macronutrients.

What happens after we have burned through that teaspoon of sugar circulating in our blood, but we are only on mile six of a half-marathon? Where do our muscles and brains find more sugar to burn? In particular, our brains constantly need glucose as fuel, or we could lose consciousness. The brain is a selfish organ that hoards much of the glucose for itself because it uses a lot of ATP (considering its importance, we'll give it a pass). Once most of the recently ingested glucose is used up—consumed by thinking up big and important ideas or that impromptu run to "work off" the calories of that yummy croissant sammy—we have to locate more of that important sugar from somewhere.

If only we had some way to store glucose in our body . . . Well, remember glycogen, those glucose molecules strewn together into a tentacled particle floating in a sea of water? Well, that glycogen lives in our muscles and liver. The liver can store about eighty grams of sugar as glycogen (about two twelve-ounce Coca-Colas' worth) at any one time. Glycogen stores are built up during the day and replenished from carbohydrates in our meals (please note that as a general principle, drinking two sugar-sweetened beverages is not a recommended way to keep the liver full of sugar). But during the night, while we are sleeping (and therefore not eating), our brains and other bodily functions still require glucose. A major source of the glucose comes from the breakdown of glycogen into a tide of glucose. The freed glucose ebbs back into our veins. We might burn through about half to three-quarters of the liver's glycogen during one night's sleep. Likewise, when we are active or haven't eaten recently, our body says, "Hey, break down some glycogen into glucose, because we need fuel to keep going." When we go for a walk or a run, we break down the glycogen in our muscles so that they have energy to move. But there's only so much glycogen stored in the muscles and liver, and that gets used up quickly.

Now let's say you're still running that half-marathon. The brain says, "What's up with this? I need more energy!" But now we're out of glycogen, and it's still a few miles to the next rest stop, and eventually lunch.

Fat to the rescue! Or, um, wait ... As you'll recall, I mentioned that the brain doesn't burn fatty acids, that it needs glucose to function, and that running burns through glucose faster. How then do we keep our brains functioning? Since sugars like glucose and fructose can be used to make fat, then maybe it is possible to reverse the process and turn a fatty acid back into glucose? Unfortunately, the short answer is "No, our bodies cannot convert fat directly into glucose."

So, while our muscles can burn either fat or glucose, the brain needs glucose. Luckily our bodies can quickly remake new glucose, even when we have run out of glycogen. This is because we have a liver—our beautiful, underappreciated liver—where glucose is made in a process called "gluconeogenesis." It's a complicated word, even more so than ATP, but it makes some logical sense. It comes from the linking of three parts: "gluco" = sugar; "neo" = new; "genesis" = coming into being. Literally, the birthing of new sugar. This occurs when other molecules like lactate (which is from partially digested glucose) or glycerol (released when we break down triglycerides to free up fatty acids) are pasted together to make new glucose. Gluconeogenesis requires energy in the form of ATP for the birthing process. This creates a seeming paradox, since it wouldn't make sense to burn glucose to make ATP, to then make more glucose! Here's the trick the liver figured out: It can burn fat in the mitochondrial furnace to make the ATP, and also use the mitochondria as a factory to start stitching together the smaller precursor pieces back into glucose. It burns up some of our stored fat to recombine other molecules like lactate, glycerol, and amino acids to "give birth" to that sugar. Here's to our mitochondria!

Hooray! We're on mile seven of that half-marathon. Our endurance muscles are quite good at burning fat to fuel the run, but our brains still need fuel. In our haste, we forgot to tuck a Clif Bar into our pocket before we left home. The brain is struggling. The liver is aware of this and, in addition to making glucose, it can convert some of the fatty acids into a hybrid molecule that is part fat and part sugar, called ketones, that the brain can also use. Because of this organization we can simultaneously burn fat and glucose while making ATP, new glucose, and ketones, all at the same time. It's a question of how much we do of each process—and that depends on whether we've eaten and what activity we're doing. If we're running, we're firing on all cylinders.

Let's take this imaginary 13.1-mile run that we just completed (congratulations!). Along with energy from our breakfast, we started with some glycogen stores left over from last night's dinner. We'll add to that some gluconeogenesis powered by fatty acids. Maybe we'll tip into ketone territory at mile 10 or so, also supported by fatty acids. But once we're home, have showered, had a banana with peanut butter, and are driving to dinner, our trusty mitochondria can continue to make ATP so we can push down on the gas pedal and wave at our neighbors.

54　*Babies need a lot of fat*

You may have heard of another type of fat besides white adipose, referred to as brown fat. Some other mammals, like mice, have a lot of brown fat, which helps maintain their body temperature. But humans have very little. We have it as babies, but we lose it over time. We don't know exactly why we shed our brown fat as we grow, but that's what happens. So as humans, not mice, we mainly have white adipose tissue, which we'll refer to as fat tissue or adipose tissue from here on out.

54　*adipose (fat) tissue is essential*

We store our fat in all the familiar places: our butt cheeks, our cherubic facial cheeks, our breasts, our love handles, our hips. It would be easy to think that we only store fat just below the surface of our skin, in all the places we can see it when we're looking at ourselves in the mirror. What we see then, in our bumps and lumps, is the subcutaneous fat.

But we also store fat in other places. Our bodies are very creative—they are not going to miss a nook or cranny that might fit a little more energy storage. One of these internal stores of fat is called visceral fat, and it's deposited in our abdomen and wrapped around our organs. There's a subset of visceral fat, omental fat, which acts like a flap that covers the organs and serves as a cushion. Some fat around our organs is helpful. It protects them, like cellular Bubble Wrap.

56 *when we store extra fat in our liver, muscles, and pancreas, it's more likely that we'll develop diabetes*

You may have heard of a fatty liver, where excess fat deposition into individual liver cells causes them to accumulate multiple smaller lipid droplets. In that case, the liver's "wiring" gets confused and it starts to make too much sugar (the excess gluconeogenesis contributing to diabetes). It can get inflamed and start to scar the liver (causing fibrosis). Too much injury can lead to cirrhosis or even liver cancer. Yikes! Because the process is often silent or painless, a lot of liver injury can occur before we, or our doctors, realize it.

Fatty acids can be absorbed from our gut after a meal of a Chicago-style hot dog or a creamy ice-cream-based milkshake. Fatty acids can enter our blood to travel normally to, or in between, different organs like adipose, the liver, and muscles. In extreme cases there is a problem storing these triglycerides, and they accumulate in the blood so much that it can become yellowish in color and turn solid and butter-like if chilled. This can lead to accumulation of fat in some of our immune cells in the skin, causing bumps (eruptive xanthomas), cardiovascular disease, or even severe, painful pancreatitis. Not good.

Our muscles can store fat too. Lipid droplets can be stored in muscle cells to provide a source of energy needed for movement. But this reservoir can also get overloaded and make the cells no longer responsive to take up glucose (termed "insulin resistance"). This condition can be an important contributor to the development of type 2 diabetes.

Chapter 3

61 *this study taught us that our body adjusts how much energy it burns based on whether it perceives us to be above or below where our fat stores were at baseline*

Dr. Kevin Hall and colleagues conducted another pivotal study investigating the metabolic response to rigorous physical activity and caloric restriction on *The Biggest Loser* TV show (the show was unfortunately quite fat-shaming). What these researchers found in the *Biggest Loser* study (2016) was that the people who ate the least lost the most weight but that the amount of weight lost was not related to the amount of exercise. Then six years later on average the participants had gained back two-thirds of the weight they had lost (which means that they maintained one-third of the weight they had lost, still a good amount of weight loss), but they had persistent metabolic adaptation, meaning that their metabolic rate remained lower than where they started. There are studies that have not found this to be the case, so other factors likely play into metabolic adaptation and continued research is needed to further our understanding. Nevertheless, this was an important finding informing us about how our bodies may conserve energy in the setting of weight loss.

73   *Where do the nearly 600,000 extra calories go?*

There are 3,500 kcals worth of energy stored in 1 pound of fat (the molecule). This has led to a frequent misinterpretation that all one would have to do to lose a pound of stored fat (the tissue) in our body is restrict the diet by 500 kcals a day for a week. This would be an incorrect interpretation because the body varies its efficiency and its activity levels in order to control the amount of fat (the tissue) that is stored in our body. The 600,000 kcal difference between what we eat and what we actually need if it were stored as fat would equate to 171 pounds in a year! The reason our weight goes up only 1 to 2 pounds a year is because of metabolic adaptation—the brain controlling how efficient our bodies are. The body wastes the vast majority of that excess energy to help maintain our energy stores at a certain level.

Chapter 4

85   *but it is more complex than that*

An important thing to know is that the body fat set point, or Enough Point, is not set by just one region of the brain. Although we don't know on a molecular level how it is set, we do at least have an idea of the various parts of the brain that are involved.

We used to think there was just the hypothalamus, the homeostasis or balance-regulating part of the brain: the part that controls hunger and satiety. But we don't eat just when we're hungry. We know now that there are hedonic (limbic—reward motivation and emotion) regions of the brain that are active. We eat for pleasure. We eat when we're stressed. We eat when we're happy. We eat for comfort. And finally, there are executive, decision-making regions of the brain (the prefrontal cortex). This is what makes us humans, helps us make conscious decisions and choices. These three regions of the brain (homeostatic, hedonic, and executive) all communicate with each other and regulate our brains' response to all those external inputs—like hormones, like food cues—and regulate how much energy our bodies want to store.

93   *There is even a Food Noise Questionnaire*
Over the years, my patients have shared many similar stories of food noise—each a bit different, all with the exhaustion that comes from battling their own biology. To better quantify this, researchers at the Pennington Biomedical Research Center, in collaboration with other scientists, produced a Food Noise Questionnaire (FNQ) in 2024. The FNQ is free for clinicians and researchers to use with citation. It asks the respondents to rate how much they agree with the following statements:

1. "I find myself constantly thinking about food throughout the day."

2. "My thoughts about food feel uncontrollable."

3. "I spend too much time thinking about food."

4. "My thoughts about food have negative effects on me and/or my life."

5. "My thoughts about food distract me from what I need to do."

The questionnaire is now a tool that researchers can begin to use in their research to better quantify food noise.

Chapter 5

100 *officially called obesity a "disease" in a publication*
"Corpulency [obesity], when in an extraordinary degree, may be reckoned a disease, as it in some measure obstructs the free exercise of the animal functions; and hath a tendency to shorten life, by paving the way to dangerous distempers [illnesses]."

101 *myxedema (a very rare*
Myxedema coma is a very rare but life-threatening result of extremely severe hypothyroidism.

101 *despite opposition from academic physicians*
It was also noted as a negative effect that excess thyroid hormone increased protein catabolism and therefore loss of lean body mass, so loss of muscle.

101 *cannot be blamed for the obesity epidemic*
As we learn more, and how to target receptors more specifically, there may be potential other uses by targeting certain thyroid hormone receptors. This has been done for the treatment of fatty liver with inflammation and scarring, with a new medication that targets thyroid hormone receptor beta and does not result in weight reduction.

101 *a chemical compound called DNP (dinitrophenol)*
DNP, dinitrophenol, was found serendipitously to decrease weight even in people without obesity. It was noted during WWI that factory workers in France who were preparing the chemical compound DNP in munitions factories were losing weight. In 1931, a Stanford pharmacologist got wind of this and tested DNP in animals. He found that DNP could induce weight loss, but had a very narrow therapeutic window—meaning that the difference in dose between what would cause weight loss and the dose that killed the animals was very small. So, with DNP that window was very narrow, meaning it was difficult for it to work without causing dangerous effects, including death.

Even as DNP was being evaluated in the early 1930s, there were three reported deaths, and other problems such as cataracts were found. It is estimated that over two thousand people lost their sight or developed neuropathy (nerve damage or malfunction), and still more people died. DNP works through mitochondrial uncoupling. Basically, that means that in the setting of DNP the powerhouses of the cell become inefficient and leak or waste energy, creating extra heat, so the body ends up burning off more energy by increasing metabolic rate—but at what cost? Unfortunately, the burning off of energy causes people to get hyperthermia (a fever but with no virus or infection causing it). By 1935, the American Medical Association (AMA) found that DNP was too hazardous for use. When FDA laws were updated in 1938, the FDA had the authority to ban DNP and did so.

106 *Orlistat (brand name Xenical and Alli)*
Even with reducing the amount of absorbed fat by 30%, the effects of orlistat are rather modest. That's because it does not work in the brain! Since it does not lower the Enough Point, the body finds other ways to ensure an adequate energy supply. So, given that your body is supersmart, what does it do? It compensates! You may eat more or become more energy efficient. Today, orlistat is sometimes used as part of the regimen to treat obesity in folks who have constipation (perhaps as a side effect of another medicine), and for this reason it can be a helpful addition. That way a few extra pounds are lost while constipation is mitigated.

108 *Metformin ... has been used*
Metformin helps prevent type 2 diabetes in people who have prediabetes and is also used to treat patients with PCOS (polycystic ovarian syndrome), though it is not FDA approved for either indication. Indeed, as in the case of metformin, it is worth noting that 12–38% of the medications prescribed in the United States are done so off-label.

113 *When people with congenital leptin deficiency*
The fact that the signal was a hormone (leptin) that came from adipocytes (fat cells) and was proportional to the amount of fat in the body radically changed the perspective and attitudes of scientists and clinicians.

Human leptin deficiency is extremely uncommon. Complete deficiency is estimated to occur in one per every ten to twenty million people and results in severe obesity beginning in infancy. As with many common diseases, it is the rare form of obesity that actually helped us begin to understand the physiology (biology) better. Individuals with leptin deficiency lack the signal (leptin) that informs various nuclei in their brains that they are storing adequate amounts of energy. Because these individuals lack the signal, they continue to gain weight and develop severe obesity even in infancy. Because their brains continue to think they are starving and living as far below their Enough Point as possible, they are extremely hungry at all times of the day and night. Because one part of the circuit is broken, the other parts of the circuit try as hard as possible to get more energy into the body.

Leptin is an unusual type of signal that is most important when it is low or missing. It informs our brains of long-term energy stores (fat tissue). So, when leptin is missing (or cannot be sensed, as is the case with leptin receptor deficiency), people gain weight because the brain thinks the body is starving to death.

119 *Enter the hormones: GLP-1 and GIP*
Numerous pivotal discoveries about the GLP-1 hormone were made by scientists who had been working in this space for decades, including Joel Habener, Svetlana Mojsov, Daniel Drucker, Lotte Bjerre Knudsen, Jens Holst, Matthias Tschöp, Richard DiMarchi, and many, many more. It literally took an international village to figure this out! What did the hormone do? How could it be made to last longer in the body? (Native human GLP-1 is broken down in just a few minutes in our bodies.) Where did it act in the body? (Turns out all over the body, including the brain.)

Chapter 6

132 *The media frenzy*
Even though the manuscript was published, the FDA had not yet approved tirzepatide for obesity treatment (it had been FDA approved for type 2 diabetes treatment in May 2022), and it would still be a while before it made its way to the pharmacies. After the publication of that study, perhaps fueled by emergence out of COVID, the world became much more interested in semaglutide (Ozempic and Wegovy), which had been FDA approved for obesity the year prior (2021).

Chapter 7

165 *not only longer but better*

The positive impact of starting exercise alongside a medication has been demonstrated with liraglutide in a study published in the *NEJM* a few years ago. These studies need to be done with newer medications as well (a great opportunity to participate in research studies!).

170 *good sleep hygiene*

In his recent book, *Why We Sleep*, Matthew Walker, PhD, details the comprehensive critical role and value of sleep and what this means for all of us.

Chapter 8

193 *additional thirty million people with diabetes*

The American Diabetes Association (ADA) definition of prediabetes is an A1c of 5.7–6.4%, impaired fasting glucose (IFG) of 100 to 125 mg/dL, or impaired glucose tolerance (IGT) of a two-hour plasma glucose from 140 to 199 mg/dL during a 75-g OGTT.

203 *other parts of her physical exam*

We also look at other characteristics that may inform us about the impact of obesity. Central adiposity (storing weight in the center of your body) is indicative of metabolic perturbations (for example, prediabetes or diabetes). Acanthosis nigricans (dark, velvety-feeling skin on the neck) is seen in people with higher insulin levels, especially children and adolescents. When someone comes in for an initial visit for obesity and they have gained weight very quickly (such as sixty pounds in three months), we also look for signs of other conditions, such as Cushing's syndrome (a disease of cortisol excess), which can be caused by a very rare cortisol-secreting tumor in the body or by chronic oral steroids, also called corticosteroids, used as a treatment for other diseases, such as chronic obstructive pulmonary disease, or COPD. Remember, medications that we as health care providers may give you for other illnesses (various mood medications for depression, beta-blockers for high blood pressure, insulin for diabetes) may also cause weight gain and are a common contributor to the development of obesity. Some signs of Cushing's syndrome include wide purple stretch marks (called striae) and a pad of fat tissue on the back of the neck. On labs we look for signs of other problems to make sure we are not missing other diseases or medical conditions.

Chapter 10

234　*help preserve muscle mass*

The degree of muscle loss we are seeing with the NuSH-based medications is not different from the muscle loss we see with bariatric surgery or caloric restriction. People with obesity have more muscle mass than people who do not have obesity (they have more weight to carry against gravity) so the lean muscle mass loss is proportional to what we would expect with other interventions. The important factor to consider is muscle function: how well our muscles, and therefore our bodies, work to help us move.

References

Preface

Akram, D. S., A. V. Astrup, T. Atinmo, et al. "Obesity: Preventing and Managing the Global Epidemic." *WHO Technical Report Series*, no. 894 (2000), i–xii, 1–253.

Introduction

Jastreboff, A. M., R. Sinha, C. Lacadie, D. M. Small, R. S. Sherwin, and M. N. Potenza. "Neural Correlates of Stress- and Food Cue-Induced Food Craving in Obesity: Association with Insulin Levels." *Diabetes Care* 36, no. 2 (Feb 2013): 394–402.

Jastreboff, A. M., R. Sinha, J. Arora, et al. "Altered Brain Response to Drinking Glucose and Fructose in Obese Adolescents." *Diabetes* 65, no. 7 (Jul 2016): 1929–39.

Zhang, Y., R. Proenca, M. Maffei, M. Barone, L. Leopold, and J. M. Friedman. "Positional Cloning of the Mouse Obese Gene and Its Human Homologue." *Nature* 372, no. 6505 (Dec 1994): 425–32.

Chapter 1

Michele Yeun, M. "Health Complications of Obesity: 224 Obesity-Associated Comorbidities from a Mechanistic Perspective." *Gastroenterology Clinics of North America* 52, no. 2 (2023): 363–80.

Puhl, R. M. "Weight Stigma and Barriers to Effective Obesity Care." *Gastroenterology Clinics of North America* 52, no. 2 (Jun 2023): 417–28.

Chapter 2

Belluz, J., and K. Hall. *Food Intelligence: The Science of How Food Both Nourishes and Harms Us.* Avery, 2025.

Bray, G. A., W. E. Heisel, A. Afshin, M. D. Jensen, et al. "The Science of Obesity Management: An Endocrine Society Scientific Statement." *Endocrine Reviews* 39, no. 2 (Apr 2018): 79–132.

Keys, A., F. Fidanza, M. J. Karvonen, N. Kimura, and H. L. Taylor. "Indices of Relative Weight and Obesity." *Journal of Chronic Diseases* 25, no. 6 (Jul 1972): 329–43.

Chapter 3

Diabetes Prevention Program Research Group. "10-Year Follow-Up of Diabetes Incidence and Weight Loss in the Diabetes Prevention Program Outcomes Study." *Lancet* 374, no. 9702 (Nov 2009): 1677–86.

Fothergill, E., J. Guo, L. Howard, et al. "Persistent Metabolic Adaptation 6 Years After 'The Biggest Loser' Competition." *Obesity* (Silver Spring) 24, no. 8 (Aug 2016): 1612–19.

Hall, K. D., A. Ayuketah, R. Brychta, et al. "Ultra-Processed Diets Cause Excess Calorie Intake and Weight Gain: An Inpatient Randomized Controlled Trial of Ad Libitum Food Intake." *Cell Metabolism* 30, no. 1 (Jul 2019): 67–77, e3.

Keesey, R. E., and M. D. Hirvonen. "Body Weight Set-Points: Determination and Adjustment." *The Journal of Nutrition* 127, no. 9 (Sep 1997): 1875S–1883S.

Kennedy, G. C. "The Role of Depot Fat in the Hypothalamic Control of Food Intake in the Rat." *Proceedings of the Royal Society B: Biological Sciences* 140, no. 901 (Jan 1953): 578–96.

Leibel, R. L., M. Rosenbaum, and J. Hirsch. "Changes in Energy Expenditure Resulting from Altered Body Weight." *The New England Journal of Medicine* 332, no. 10 (Mar 1995): 621–28.

Sumithran, P., L. A. Prendergast, E. Delbridge, K. Purcell, A. Shulkes, A. Kriketos, and J. Proietto. "Long-Term Persistence of Hormonal Adaptations to Weight Loss." *The New England Journal of Medicine* 365, no. 17 (Oct 2011): 1597–604.

Chapter 4

Bray, G. A., W. E. Heisel, A. Afshin, et al. "The Science of Obesity Management: An Endocrine Society Scientific Statement." *Endocrine Reviews* 39, no. 2 (Apr 2018): 79–132.

Diktas, H. E., M. I. Cardel, G. D. Foster, et al. "Development and Validation of the Food Noise Questionnaire." *Obesity* (Silver Spring) 33, no. 2 (Feb 2025): 289–97.

Chapter 5

Bray, G. A. "Obesity: A 100 Year Perspective." *International Journal of Obesity* 49, no. 2 (Feb 2025): 159–67.

Drucker, D. J. "Discovery of GLP-1-Based Drugs for the Treatment of Obesity." *The New England Journal of Medicine* 392, no. 6 (Feb 2025): 612–15.

Farooqi, I. S., S. A. Jebb, G. Langmack, et al. "Effects of Recombinant Leptin Therapy in a Child with Congenital Leptin Deficiency." *The New England Journal of Medicine* 341, no. 12 (Sep 1999): 879–84.

Jastreboff, A. M., L. J. Aronne, N. N. Ahmad, et al., for the SURMOUNT-1 Investigators. "Tirzepatide Once Weekly for the Treatment of Obesity." *The New England Journal of Medicine* 387, no. 3 (Jul 2022): 205–16.

Pi-Sunyer, X., A. Astrup, K. Fujioka, et al., for the SCALE Obesity and Prediabetes NN8022-1839 Study Group. "A Randomized, Controlled Trial of 3.0 mg of Liraglutide in Weight Management," *The New England Journal of Medicine* 373, no. 1 (Jul 2015): 11–22.

Sjöström, L., K. Narbro, C. D. Sjöström, et al., for the Swedish Obese Subjects Study. "Effects of Bariatric Surgery on Mortality in Swedish Obese Subjects," *The New England Journal of Medicine* 357, no. 8 (Aug 2007): 741–52.

Wilding, J. P. H., R. L. Batterham, S. Calanna, et al., for the STEP 1 Study Group. "Once-Weekly Semaglutide in Adults with Overweight or Obesity." *The New England Journal of Medicine* 384, no. 11 (Mar 2021): 989–1002.

Chapter 6

Gossmann, M., W. S. Butsch, and A. M. Jastreboff. "Treating the Chronic Disease of Obesity." *Medical Clinics of North America* 105, no. 6 (Nov 2021): 983–1016.

Jastreboff, A. M., L. J. Aronne, N. N. Ahmad, et al., for the SURMOUNT-1 Investigators. "Tirzepatide Once Weekly for the Treatment of Obesity." *The New England Journal of Medicine* 387, no. 3 (Jul 2022): 205–16.

Kaplan, L. M., K. Gudzune, J. Ard, et al. "Perceptions of Anti-Obesity Medications Among People with Obesity and Healthcare Providers in the US: Findings from the OBSERVE Study." *Obesity* (Silver Spring) 33, no. 6 (Jun 2025): 1076–86.

Chapter 7

Almandoz, J. P., T. A. Wadden, C. Tewksbury, et al. "Nutritional Considerations with Antiobesity Medications." *Obesity* (Silver Spring) 32, no. 9 (Sep 2024): 1613–31.

Aronne, L. J., D. B. Horn, C. W. le Roux, et al., for the SURMOUNT-5 Trial Investigators. "Tirzepatide as Compared with Semaglutide for the Treatment of Obesity." *The New England Journal of Medicine* 393, no. 1 (Jul 2025): 26–36.

Aronne, L. J., N. Sattar, D. B. Horn, et al. "Continued Treatment with Tirzepatide for Maintenance of Weight Reduction in Adults with Obesity: The SURMOUNT-4 Randomized Clinical Trial." *JAMA* 331, no. 1 (Jan 2024): 38–48.

Lundgren, J. R., C. Janus, S. B. K. Jensen, et al. "Healthy Weight Loss Maintenance with Exercise, Liraglutide, or Both Combined." *The New England Journal of Medicine* 384, no. 18 (May 2021): 1719–30.

Markwald, R. R., E. L. Melanson, M. R. Smith, et al. "Impact of Insufficient Sleep on Total Daily Energy Expenditure, Food Intake, and Weight Gain." *PNAS* 110, no. 14 (Apr 2013): 5695–700.

Ryan, D. H., and S. R. Yockey. "Weight Loss and Improvement in Comorbidity: Differences at 5%, 10%, 15%, and Over." *Current Obesity Reports* 6 (2017): 187–94.

Sinha, R., and A. M. Jastreboff. "Stress as a Common Risk Factor for Obesity and Addiction." *Biological Psychiatry* 73, no. 9 (May 2013): 827–35.

Tanofsky-Kraff, M., N. A. Schvey, R. O. Pashby, and N. L. Burke. *The New Food Fight: How the Weight Management and Eating Disorder Fields Became So Divided and What We Can Do About It*. Oxford University Press, 2025.

Wilding, J. P. H., R. L. Batterham, M. Davies, et al. "Weight Regain and Cardiometabolic Effects After Withdrawal of Semaglutide: The STEP 1

Trial Extension." *Diabetes, Obesity and Metabolism* 24, no. 8 (Aug 2022): 1553–64.

Chapter 8

Aronne, L. J., K. D. Hall, J. M. Jakicic, et al. "Describing the Weight-Reduced State: Physiology, Behavior, and Interventions." *Obesity* (Silver Spring) 29, suppl. 1 (Apr 2021): S9–S24.

Bjornstad, P., K. L. Drews, S. Caprio, et al., for the TODAY Study Group. "Long-Term Complications in Youth-Onset Type 2 Diabetes." *The New England Journal of Medicine* 385, no. 5 (Jul 2021): 416–26.

Bliddal, H., H. Bays, S. Czernichow, et al., for the STEP 9 Study Group. "Once-Weekly Semaglutide in Persons with Obesity and Knee Osteoarthritis." *The New England Journal of Medicine* 391, no. 17 (Oct 2024): 1573–83.

Gossmann, M., W. S. Butsch, and A. M. Jastreboff. "Treating the Chronic Disease of Obesity." *Medical Clinics of North America* 105, no. 6 (Nov 2021): 983–1016.

Jastreboff, A. M., C. W. le Roux, A. Stefanski, et al., for the SURMOUNT-1 Investigators. "Tirzepatide for Obesity Treatment and Diabetes Prevention." *The New England Journal of Medicine* 392, no. 10 (Mar 2025): 958–71.

Kosiborod, M. N., S. Z. Abildstrøm, B. A. Borlaug, et al., for the STEP-HFpEF Trial Committees and Investigators. "Semaglutide in Patients with Heart Failure with Preserved Ejection Fraction and Obesity." *The New England Journal of Medicine* 389, no. 12 (Aug 2023): 1069–84.

Lam, C. S. P., A. Rodriguez, A. Aminian, et al. "Tirzepatide for Reduction of Morbidity and Mortality in Adults with Obesity: Rationale and Design of the SURMOUNT-MMO Trial." *Obesity* (Silver Spring) 33, no. 9 (Sep 2025): 1645–56.

Lincoff, A. M., K. Brown-Frandsen, H. M. Colhoun, et al., for the SELECT Trial Investigators. "Semaglutide and Cardiovascular Outcomes in Obesity without Diabetes." *The New England Journal of Medicine* 389, no. 24 (Dec 2023): 2221–32.

Malhotra, A., J. Bednarik, S. Chakladar, et al. "Tirzepatide for the Treatment of Obstructive Sleep Apnea: Rationale, Design, and Sample Baseline Characteristics of the SURMOUNT - OSA Phase 3 Trial." *Contemporary Clinical Trials* 141, no. 107516 (Jun 2024).

References

Packer, M., M. R. Zile, C. M. Kramer, et al., for the SUMMIT Trial Study Group. "Tirzepatide for Heart Failure with Preserved Ejection Fraction and Obesity." *The New England Journal of Medicine* 392, no. 5 (Jan 2025): 427–37.

Weghuber, D., T. Barrett, M. Barrientos-Pérez, et al., for the STEP TEENS Investigators. "Once-Weekly Semaglutide in Adolescents with Obesity." *The New England Journal of Medicine* 387, no. 24 (Dec 2022): 2245–57.

Chapter 9

Aronne, L. J., D. B. Horn, C. W. le Roux, et al., for the SURMOUNT-5 Trial Investigators. "Tirzepatide as Compared with Semaglutide for the Treatment of Obesity." *The New England Journal of Medicine* 393, no. 1 (Jul 2025): 26–36.

Bjerre Knudsen, L., L. W. Madsen, S. Andersen, et al. "Glucagon-Like Peptide-1 Receptor Agonists Activate Rodent Thyroid C-Cells Causing Calcitonin Release and C-Cell Proliferation." *Endocrinology* 151, no. 4 (Apr 2010): 1473–86.

Drucker, D. J. "Efficacy and Safety of GLP-1 Medicines for Type 2 Diabetes and Obesity." *Diabetes Care* 47, no. 11 (Nov 2024): 1873–88.

European Medicines Agency. "Meeting Highlights from the Pharmacovigilance Risk Assessment Committee (PRAC) 8-11 April 2024," April 12, 2024.

Gorgojo-Martínez, J. J., P. Mezquita-Raya, J. Carretero-Gómez, et al. "Clinical Recommendations to Manage Gastrointestinal Adverse Events in Patients Treated with GLP-1 Receptor Agonists: A Multidisciplinary Expert Consensus." *Journal of Clinical Medicine* 12, no. 1 (Dec 2022): 145.

Jastreboff, A. M., L. J. Aronne, N. N. Ahmad, et al., for the SURMOUNT-1 Investigators. "Tirzepatide Once Weekly for the Treatment of Obesity." *The New England Journal of Medicine* 387, no. 3 (Jul 2022): 205–16.

Kerem, L., and J. Stokar. "Risk of Suicidal Ideation or Attempts in Adolescents with Obesity Treated with GLP1 Receptor Agonists." *JAMA Pediatrics* 178, no. 12 (Dec 2024): 1307–15.

US Food and Drug Administration. "Update on FDA's Ongoing Evaluation of Reports of Suicidal Thoughts or Actions in Patients Taking a Certain Type of Medicines Approved for Type 2 Diabetes and Obesity: Preliminary Evaluation Does Not Suggest a Causal Link." FDA Drug Safety Communication, January 11, 2024. Updated January 30, 2024.

Wilding, J. P. H., R. L. Batterham, S. Calanna, et al., for the STEP 1 Study Group. "Once-Weekly Semaglutide in Adults with Overweight or Obesity." *The New England Journal of Medicine* 384, no. 11 (Mar 2021): 989–1002.

Chapter 10

Drucker, D. J. "GLP-1-Based Therapies for Diabetes, Obesity and Beyond." *Nature Reviews Drug Discovery* 24 (2025): 631–50.

Garvey, W. T., M. Blüher, C. K. Osorto Contreras, et al., for the REDEFINE 1 Study Group. "Coadministered Cagrilintide and Semaglutide in Adults with Overweight or Obesity." *The New England Journal of Medicine* 393, no. 7 (Aug 2025): 635–47.

Jastreboff, A. M., D. H. Ryan, H. E. Bays, et al., for the MariTide Phase 2 Obesity Trial Investigators. "Once-Monthly Maridebart Cafraglutide for the Treatment of Obesity—A Phase 2 Trial." *The New England Journal of Medicine* 393, no. 9 (Sep 2025): 843–57.

Jastreboff, A. M., L. M. Kaplan, J. P. Frías, et al., for the Retatrutide Phase 2 Obesity Trial Investigators. "Triple-Hormone-Receptor Agonist Retatrutide for Obesity - A Phase 2 Trial." *The New England Journal of Medicine* 389, no. 6 (Aug 2023): 514–26.

Knop, F. K., V. R. Aroda, R. D. do Vale, et al. "Oral Semaglutide 50 mg Taken Once Per Day in Adults with Overweight or Obesity (OASIS 1): A Randomised, Double-Blind, Placebo-Controlled, Phase 3 Trial." *Lancet* 402, no. 10403 (Aug 2023): 705–19.

le Roux, C. W., O. Steen, K. J. Lucas, E. Startseva, A. Unseld, and A. M. Hennige. "Glucagon and GLP-1 Receptor Dual Agonist Survodutide for Obesity: A Randomised, Double-Blind, Placebo-Controlled, Dose-Finding Phase 2 Trial." *Lancet Diabetes Endocrinology* 12, no. 3 (Mar 2024): 162–73.

Melson, E., U. Ashraf, D. Papamargaritis, and M. J. Davies. "What Is the Pipeline for Future Medications for Obesity?" *International Journal of Obesity* 49, no. 3 (Mar 2025): 433–51.

Wharton, S., L. J. Aronne, A. Stefanski, et al., for the ATTAIN-1 Trial Investigators. "Orforglipron, an Oral Small-Molecule GLP-1 Receptor Agonist for Obesity Treatment." *The New England Journal of Medicine* (Sep 2025).